Clinical Parasitology

Clinical Parasitology
A Handbook for Medical Practitioners and Microbiologists

Harsha Sheorey MD, FRCPA
John Walker BSc, MSc, PhD
Beverley-Ann Biggs FRACP, PhD, FRCP, FACTM

MELBOURNE UNIVERSITY PRESS

MELBOURNE UNIVERSITY PRESS
PO Box 278, Carlton South, Victoria 3053, Australia
info@mup.unimelb.edu.au
www.mup.com.au

First published 2000
Text © Harsha Sheorey, John Walker and Beverley-Ann Biggs 2000
Design and typography © Melbourne University Press 2000

Designed and typeset by Melbourne University Press
Printed in Australia by Impact Printing, Brunswick, Victoria

National Library of Australia Cataloguing-in-Publication entry

Sheorey, Harsha, 1956– .
   Clinical parasitology: a handbook for medical
   practitioners and microbiologists
   Includes index.
   ISBN 0 522 84834 6.
   1. Parasites—Handbooks manuals, etc. 2. Parasitic
   diseases—Handbooks manuals, etc. 3. Parasitology. I.
   Walker, John Charles, 1938– . II. Biggs, Beverley-Ann.
   III. Title.
616.96

Publication of this work was sponsored by the Victorian Infectious Diseases Reference Laboratory and the Victorian Infectious Diseases Service.

Every effort has been made to ensure that the information in this book is accurate at the time of publication. The authors are not responsible for the effects of subsequent change.

Foreword

Scarcely a year goes by without the implication of another parasite in the causation of human disease, often with disastrous consequences for an individual or a community. Practitioners of infectious diseases and other specialties in internal medicine, and microbiologists need to be aware of the range of parasites that can cause disease in normal and immunocompromised hosts. This has become more important in recent years as an increasing number of Australians travel abroad and risk infections from various exotic parasites. This handbook provides a succinct and practical guide to the diagnosis and management of parasitic diseases and will be a valuable guide for those practising at both the hospital and primary health care level.

The Victorian Infectious Diseases Reference Laboratory in Melbourne (VIDRL) and the Centre for Infectious Diseases and Microbiology in Sydney (CIDM) have well-earned reputations for excellence as referral centres for unusual pathogens from all over Australia. Previously located at Fairfield Hospital, VIDRL continues to provide a key reference role as part of the North Western Health Care campus, where continuing collaboration exists with clinicians formerly located at Fairfield Hospital who are now working with the Victorian Infectious Diseases Service. CIDM is linked with the University of Sydney and has worked closely with clinicians at Westmead Hospital for many years.

In this excellent handbook of clinical parasitology, the authors attempt to provide the elements of basic clinical parasitology with aspects of microscopic and serological diagnosis and treatment. They have achieved these aims admirably and have produced a book that will be relevant for clinical practitioners as well as laboratory scientists.

Graham V. Brown

MB BS, MPH, MRACP, FRACP, PhD, FAFPHM, FACTM

James Stewart Professor of Medicine, University of Melbourne

Head of the Victorian Infectious Diseases Service, Royal Melbourne Hospital

Contents

Foreword by Graham V. Brown   *v*

Acknowledgements   *xi*

Acanthamoeba spp.   1

Ancylostoma spp.
    A. braziliense   4
    A. caninum   4

Angiostrongylus spp.
    A. cantonensis   6
    A. costaricensis   7

Anisakis spp.   9

Ascaris lumbricoides   11

Babesia microti   13

Balantidium coli   15

Blastocystis hominis   17

Capillaria philippinensis   19

Cryptosporidium parvum   21

Cyclospora cayetanensis   23

Dientamoeba fragilis   25

Diphyllobothrium latum   27

Dirofilaria immitis   29

Dracunculus medinensis   31

Echinococcus spp.
    E. granulosus   33
    E. multilocularis   35

Entamoeba histolytica   37

Enterobius vermicularis   40

Fasciola spp.
    F. gigantica   42
    F. hepatica   42

Fasciolopsis buski and *Brachylaima* spp.   44

Giardia duodenalis   46

Contents

Gnathostoma spinigerum   48

Hookworms
  Ancylostoma duodenale   50
  Necator americanus   50

Hymenolepis nana   52

Isospora belli   53

Leishmania spp.   55

Loa loa   59

Maggots (larval forms of flies or fleas)   61

Mansonella spp.
  M. ozzardi   63
  M. perstans   64
  M. streptocerca   65

Microsporidia   67

Naegleria fowleri   70

Onchocerca volvulus   72

Opisthorchis (Clonorchis) spp.   74

Paragonimus spp.
  P. mexicanus   76
  P. westermani   76

Pediculus spp.
  P. capitis   78
  P. humanis (corporis)   79

Phthirus pubis   81

Plasmodium spp.   83
  P. falciparum   83
  P. vivax, P. ovale and *P. malariae*   86

Pneumocystis carinii   90

Sarcoptes scabei   93

Schistosoma spp.   95
  S. haematobium   95
  S. intercalatum   97
  S. japonicum   98
  S. mansoni   99
  S. mekongi   100

Spirometra spp.   102

Strongyloides stercoralis   104

Taenia spp.
   T. saginata — 107
   T. solium — 108
   Cysticercosis — 109

Toxocara spp.
   T. canis — 112
   T. cati — 112

Toxoplasma gondii — 114

Trichinella spp.
   T. pseudospiralis — 118
   T. spiralis — 118

Trichomonas vaginalis — 120

Trichostrongylus spp. — 122

Trichuris trichiura — 123

Trypanosoma spp.
   T. brucei (gambiense and *rhodesiense)* — 125
   T. cruzi — 127

Wuchereria bancrofti and *Brugia* spp. — 130

Appendices
1 Classification and biology of parasites — 133
2 Geographical distribution of parasites — 139
3 Clinical presentations in parasitic infections — 140
4 Antiparasitic drugs and parasites for which they are used — 141
5 Access to unapproved drugs via the Special Access Scheme — 146
6 Useful addresses and contacts — 147

Glossary — 150

References — 153

Index — 160

Acknowledgements

The information presented here was collected from various sources including *Mandell, Douglas and Bennett's Principles and Practice of Infectious Diseases*,[1] *Diagnostic Medical Parasitology*,[2] *Manson's Tropical Diseases*,[3] *Therapeutic Guidelines: Antibiotic*,[4] the Division of Parasitic Diseases, Centers for Disease Control, recent journal articles, and our own work in progress. A limited list of references, mainly written by Australian authors, has been compiled to credit the excellent input that Australians continue to have in the area of clinical parasitology. We would especially like to thank Professor Stephen Locarnini, Dr David Leslie and Dr Geoff Hogg at the Victorian Infectious Diseases Reference Laboratory (VIDRL) for supporting our work in clinical parasitology, Dr Norbet Ryan for his excellent photography, Joe Manitta and Dr John Slavin for lending photographs from their collection, Jenny Leydon for providing information on serological testing, Drs Maria Yates and Allen Yung, Professors John Hayman and Graham Brown for helpful comments, and Julie Doig and Virginia de Crespigny for preparation of the manuscript. As well, Julie Lord at the Drug Information Centre, St Vincent's Hospital Pharmacy has provided information on the formulations of anti-parasitic drugs available in Australia. In particular we thank Drs Joc Forsyth and Alan Street for critically reviewing the manuscript. We are indebted to VIDRL and the Victorian Infectious Diseases Service (VIDS) for sponsoring the publication of this book.

Dr Sheorey is currently working as a Fellow in Microbiology at St Vincent's Hospital, Melbourne. Dr Walker is a Senior Lecturer in the Department of Medicine, University of Sydney, and is Director of the Parasitology Section, Institute of Clinical Pathology and Medical Research at Westmead Hospital, Sydney. Dr Biggs is a Senior Lecturer in the Department of Medicine, University of Melbourne, and an Infectious Diseases physician and Clinical Parasitologist with VIDRL and VIDS.

Acanthamoeba spp.

Protozoa: free-living freshwater amoebae

CNS and skin

LIFE CYCLE AND EPIDEMIOLOGY
These organisms are ubiquitous in lakes, soil, dust, tap water, swimming pools, and heating and air-conditioning units. Entry is usually through the skin, sinuses or lungs with subsequent haematogenous spread to the CNS. There is a worldwide distribution.

CLINICAL NOTES

Granulomatous amoebic encephalitis (GAE) is a rare, slowly progressive neurological disease, usually in the debilitated or immunosuppressed patient (including AIDS patients with CD4 $< 0.05 \times 10^9$/L). Clinical features may be present for months and include focal neurological deficits, abnormal mental state, seizures, fever, headache, hemiparesis, meningism, visual disturbances and ataxia. Cases of GAE may rarely be caused by organisms of the genera *Hartmannella*, *Vahlkampfia* or *Balamuthia* (recently recognised potentially pathogenic leptomyxid amoebae found in the soil).

Skin lesions (disseminated nodules, plaques, ulcers or abscesses) may predate the onset of CNS disease (recently described in HIV patients).[5,6] This presentation has also been reported in an Australian child with *B. mandrillaris*.[7]

Pneumonitis may occur.

DIAGNOSIS

The diagnosis requires a tissue biopsy (skin and/or brain).

* Microscopic examination for trophozoites and cysts (no flagellate stage). Special stains and IFA are available in certain centres.

> In a counting chamber, organisms may resemble leucocytes in the CSF.

* Histological examination usually reveals amoebic granulomas containing trophozoites and cysts.
* Culture of organisms on non-nutrient agar with an overlay of *Escherichia coli* is occasionally successful.
* Most cases are diagnosed post-mortem.

TREATMENT

Amphotericin B 1 mg/kg per day iv

> Treatment is of limited or unproven efficacy.

Early treatment with intravenous pentamidine, oral fluconazole, sulfadiazine and flucytosine has also been used. Topical chlorhexidine and ketoconazole cream has been recommended for HIV patients with cutaneous lesions (pentamidine, ketoconazole, miconazole, paromomycin and flucytosine all have *in vitro* activity).[5,6]

FOLLOW UP

Monitor the clinical course.

The eye

LIFE CYCLE AND EPIDEMIOLOGY

There is a rising incidence of *Acanthamoeba* corneal infection in healthy people (> 85% are soft contact lens wearers), and after trauma (often minor) that has resulted in corneal abrasions. Organisms have been isolated from contaminated water and contact lens cleaning solutions (especially chlorine cleaning solutions). Infection is also associated with wearing lenses while swimming. There is a worldwide distribution.

CLINICAL NOTES

Acanthamoeba keratitis is most often confused with viral (especially due to Herpes simplex) keratitis and fungal keratitis. The diagnosis of herpetic keratitis in a wearer of soft contact lenses should be regarded with suspicion. Patients often present with a foreign-body-like irritation, leading to severe pain, photophobia, conjunctivitis and blurred vision. Early signs of keratitis include punctate keratopathy, pseudodendrites, and epithelial and subepithelial infiltrates. Corneal ring infiltrates and corneal ulcers occur late in the clinical course. Occasionally cataracts, and more rarely hypopyon, raised intraocular pressure and nodular scleritis, are observed. Secondary bacterial infections may occur. Remissions and relapses occur. Keratitis may rarely be caused by organisms of the genera *Hartmannella* and *Vahlkampfia*.

DIAGNOSIS

- Slit lamp examination is essential.
- Microscopic examination of a corneal scraping or biopsy for trophozoites and cysts using a Calcofluor white stain.
- Wet mount to detect motility (see Plate 1).
- Culture on non-nutrient agar with an overlay growth of *E. coli* should be attempted, although it has a low sensitivity.

TREATMENT

Medical therapy alone may be curative if initiated early (i.e. if symptoms have been present for less than 6 weeks).[8]

A combination of **propamidine** and **polyhexamethylene biguanide** (PHMB) with or without **neosporin** and **chlorhexidine** is used topically.

Non-steroidal anti-inflammatory drugs are useful for controlling pain. Systemic corticosteroids may be required in severe cases of scleritis. An alternative combination of **itraconazole** and topical **miconazole** is also used.[9]

> The regimen is complex and ophthalmological consultation should be sought.

Surgical debridement and/or corneal grafting is often required, especially if symptoms have been present for more than 6 weeks.

Keratoplasty is indicated if the condition is refractory to medical treatment after 6 weeks, but before scleral invasion has occurred.

FOLLOW UP

Regular slit lamp examination to monitor the response to therapy.

DRUG AVAILABILITY IN AUSTRALIA

Amphotericin B *Fungizone* intravenous: 50 mg vials

Chlorhexidine Chlorhexidine aqueous irrigations (0.02%): prepared by pharmacy

Itraconazole *Sporonox:* 100 mg caps

Miconazole *Daktarin:* no longer available in Australia

Neomycin–polymyxin B–gramicidin *Neosporin* solution

PHMB 0.02% (polyhexamethylene biguanide) Prepared by pharmacy

Propamidine 0.1% *Brolene* eye drops

Sulfadiazine *Sulphadiazine* injection BP: 4 mL vials (1 g/4 mL)

Ancylostoma braziliense
Ancylostoma caninum

Tissue nematodes: animal hookworms (dog or cat)

LIFE CYCLE AND EPIDEMIOLOGY

Larvae of hookworms that infect animals can penetrate the human skin, but do not develop any further. Infection is acquired from soil contaminated by infective (filariform) larvae. The portal of entry is via the mouth or intact skin.

Infection is most common in children and is widespread in tropical regions, especially along the coast on sandy beaches. It is an occupational hazard for gardeners, construction workers and plumbers. Children playing in sandpits may be at risk.

There is a high incidence of eosinophilic enteritis (segmental eosinophilic inflammation of the gastrointestinal tract) among dog owners in Northern Queensland, which appears to be due to *A. caninum* infection.[10,11] Almost all cases reported so far have been in warm, humid areas and have had a close association with dogs.

CLINICAL NOTES

Cutaneous larva migrans (CLM) or 'creeping eruption' manifests as serpiginous, reddened, elevated, pruritic skin lesions that usually occur around the feet, but also on the hands or buttocks.[12] Linear tracks progress several millimetres each day. The illness is usually self-limiting, lasting 2–8 weeks. Larvae may migrate to the lungs and cause pneumonitis. The main differential diagnoses are scabies and larva currens (see *Strongyloides stercoralis*).

Eosinophilic enteritis is characterised by abdominal pain and distension, diarrhoea, weight loss, rectal bleeding and eosinophilia. The illness is self-limiting, but is responsive to mebendazole and albendazole.

DIAGNOSIS

- CLM is usually a clinical diagnosis made on the basis of the characteristic linear tracts and a history of exposure.
- Peripheral eosinophilia is common.
- Larvae are usually **not** demonstrable in skin biopsy. Larvae and eosinophils may be present in sputum in cases of pneumonitis.

- Eosinophilic enteritis has been diagnosed by finding adult *A. caninum* attached to bowel mucosa at colonoscopy.
- Serology is not currently available in Australia.

TREATMENT

For CLM:

Ivermectin 12 mg stat po (repeat treatment may be required for relapses),

or **Albendazole** 200 mg twice daily po for 3 days,

or **Thiabendazole** 25 mg/kg twice daily po (max. 3 g/day) for 2–5 days. Repeat after 2 days if active lesion persists. Side effects are common.

Topical treatment may be useful in localised CLM:

Thiabendazole 10% aqueous suspension four times daily topically (made up by hospital pharmacy). Therapy may need to be prolonged.[12]

Cryotherapy may be useful if larvae are near the surface of the skin.

For eosinophilic enterocolitis:

Mebendazole 100 mg twice daily po for 3 days,

or **Albendazole** 400 mg stat po

FOLLOW UP

Monitor the clinical response to therapy.

DRUG AVAILABILITY IN AUSTRALIA

Albendazole *Eskazole:* 400 mg tabs
            Zentel: 200 mg tabs
Ivermectin *Stromectol:* 6 mg tabs
Mebendazole *Banworm:* 100 mg tabs
            Sqworm: 100 mg tabs
            Vermox: 100 mg tabs; 100 mg/5 mL suspension
Thiabendazole *Mintezol:* 500 mg tabs

Angiostrongylus spp.

Tissue nematodes: rat lungworm

Also called *Parastrongylus* spp.

Angiostrongylus cantonensis

LIFE CYCLE AND EPIDEMIOLOGY

Adult worms reside in the pulmonary arteries of rats and other rodents. Eggs hatch in the lungs and the larvae migrate to the pharynx, are swallowed and excreted in the faeces. The parasite then develops into infective third-stage larvae in an intermediate host (snail or slug). Human disease is associated with eating undercooked snails or uncooked paratenic (i.e. transport) hosts such as prawns, crabs and frogs, or food such as unwashed leafy vegetables contaminated with molluscs. Larvae migrate to the brain and spinal cord and maturation is arrested at the young adult stage.

Gardeners, horticulturists, produce vendors and salad chefs are at greatest risk.[10,13] Children who eat snails and slugs are also at particular risk. The infection is most common in South East Asia (especially Thailand), the South Pacific (especially Tahiti) and Taiwan. It is also found in Egypt, Cuba, the Ivory Coast, Northern Australia, and has been reported as far south as Sydney.[14]

CLINICAL NOTES

The commonest clinical presentation is **eosinophilic meningitis**. The incubation period is 1–2 weeks, but may be longer. Severe headache, fever and vomiting are prominent symptoms. Stiff neck, rash, abdominal pain and malaise may occur. Neurological manifestations include seizures, paraesthesia, pain, weakness, focal deficits (especially papilloedema, extra-ocular cranial nerve palsies)[15] and, more rarely, brain abscess, coma and death. Eye involvement with visual loss, pain, iridocyclitis and retinal detachment may occur.

DIAGNOSIS

- An eosinophilic pleocytosis (> 10% of cells) is present in the CSF. Larvae are seen occasionally.

Microscopy for eosinophils in the CSF must be specifically requested.

6

- **Serology** An EIA using a semi-purified soluble extract of adult *A. cantonensis* worms as antigen is available. Assay sensitivity and specificity is unknown; however, there appears to be significant cross-reactivity with filariasis and strongyloidiasis. The specificity of the test for *A. costaricensis* is unknown.
- Perform slit lamp examination if there is a history of ocular involvement.
- Peripheral eosinophilia is common (usually > 10% of total WCC).

> Infection with *Gnathostoma spinigerum* also causes eosinophilic meningitis. Also consider cysticercosis, paragonimiasis, schistosomiasis, strongyloidiasis and trichinosis in the differential diagnosis.

TREATMENT

Surgical removal of the worm, if present in the eye, should be attempted. Repeated lumbar punctures often relieve symptoms in patients with meningitis.

> **Medical treatment is of limited or unproven efficacy.**

Mebendazole 100 mg twice daily po for 5 days,

plus **Corticosteroids** 30–60 mg/day (in severe cases with cerebral involvement).[15]

FOLLOW UP

Monitor the clinical course, peripheral eosinophil count and CSF (pleocytosis). Recovery occurs by 2 months in most patients.

Angiostrongylus costaricensis

LIFE CYCLE AND EPIDEMIOLOGY

Rats are the definitive hosts. In humans, infection is acquired by accidental ingestion of raw slugs (intermediate host) or contaminated leafy vegetables. The parasite develops in the lower small bowel and adjacent colon where degeneration of eggs and larvae cause a local inflammatory response.

There is a wide geographic distribution from the USA to Argentina. Abdominal angiostrongyliasis is most common in Costa Rica, and occurs mainly in children less than 13 years old. It is rare in Africa.

CLINICAL NOTES

Abdominal angiostrongyliasis is most common in children. It mimics appendicitis with eosinophilia. Presentation is with abdominal pain and vomiting. Surgery is often performed for suspected appendicitis. There is a RLQ mass in about 50% of cases. Differentiate from massive *Ascaris* infections.

DIAGNOSIS

- Histopathology of biopsy or excised tissue shows eosinophilic infiltration of the intestinal wall, eosinophilic vasculitis and a granulomatous reaction. Eggs and larvae can sometimes be identified.
- Peripheral leucocytosis with eosinophilia is common.
- Serology (see *A. cantonensis* for details).

TREATMENT

Most patients undergo **laparotomy** and excision of inflamed areas.

> **Medical treatment is of limited or unproven efficacy.**

Thiabendazole   25 mg/kg twice daily po for 3 days (maximum 1.5 g/day).

FOLLOW UP

Monitor the clinical course.

DRUG AVAILABILITY IN AUSTRALIA

Mebendazole   *Banworm:* 100 mg tabs
Sqworm: 100 mg tabs
Vermox: 100 mg tabs; 100 mg/5 mL suspension
Thiabendazole   *Mintezol:* 500 mg tabs

Anisakis spp.

Tissue nematodes

LIFE CYCLE AND EPIDEMIOLOGY

The adult worm lives in the stomach of large marine mammals (dolphins and whales). Eggs hatch in seawater and the free-living, second-stage larvae are ingested by small crustaceans. Third-stage larvae develop that are infective to fish and squid. Eventually, infected fish are ingested by the definitive host (marine mammals). Humans acquire the infection after eating raw or improperly cooked infected squid or marine fish such as herring, whiting or mackerel. After ingestion, the larvae penetrate the gastric and intestinal mucosa, causing the symptoms of anisakiasis.

The infection is most prevalent in Asia (especially Japan), but also wherever raw fish is eaten, as in Europe and the USA (where it has been associated with sushi bars) and the Pacific Coast of South America. It is rare in other countries and has not been reported in Australia.

CLINICAL NOTES

Sudden abdominal pain, nausea, vomiting and diarrhoea usually occur within 24–48 hours of eating the seafood meal. The larvae are large (2–3 cm long × 1 mm) and, depending on their location (gastric or intestinal), may produce symptoms that mimic peptic ulcer, appendicitis or other causes of an acute abdomen. The larvae are occasionally coughed up. Chronic symptoms of ill-health and abdominal pain, sometimes mimicking Crohn's disease, occur less commonly and may persist for several weeks to months. Intestinal masses are occasionally found and may be mistaken for an intestinal malignancy.

DIAGNOSIS

- Leucocytosis is common, but eosinophilia is usually not present.
- Observation of larvae and associated tissue inflammation on gastroscopy and microscopic identification of larva if removal is possible.
- Serology is not available in Australia and is of limited usefulness.
- Chronic intestinal anisakiasis is diagnosed by histopathological examination of tissue samples.

Anisakis spp.

Most patients improve spontaneously, but this is hastened by **surgical or endoscopic removal** of the larvae. In chronic cases, resection of the affected area is usually required to make the diagnosis and effect a cure.

Medical therapy is of unproven efficacy.

Mebendazole   200 mg twice daily po for 3 days.[16,17]

FOLLOW UP

Monitor the clinical course and WCC.

DRUG AVAILABILITY IN AUSTRALIA

Mebendazole   *Banworm:* 100 mg tabs
Sqworm: 100 mg tabs
Vermox: 100 mg tabs; 100 mg/5 mL suspension

Ascaris lumbricoides

Intestinal nematode: round worm

Infection is acquired by ingestion of eggs in contaminated soil. After hatching in the stomach and duodenum, larvae penetrate the intestinal wall and are carried via the portal, and then systemic, circulation to the lungs where they mature and migrate through the lungs into the trachea, and are coughed up and swallowed to reach the jejunum. Maturation is completed and egg production begins in 2–3 months. Adult worms can live for 1–2 years. A female may produce up to 240 000 eggs per day, which are passed in the faeces and become infectious in 2–4 weeks. Eggs may remain infectious for years.

There is a worldwide distribution (but especially in Asia, Africa and Latin America) with an estimated 1.4 billion people infected. The infection is most common in children in tropical and subtropical regions, and areas with inadequate sanitation. Occasionally, infection with the morphologically similar *A. suum* has been reported in pig-farming families.

CLINICAL NOTES

Infection is usually asymptomatic (an incidental finding in the stool or a history of passing a worm) or there are mild gastrointestinal symptoms such as abdominal pain, distension, nausea, and occasional diarrhoea. Intestinal obstruction is a complication in children with a heavy worm burden. Vomiting of worms may give a clue. Appendicular, hepatobiliary and pancreatic ascariasis is not uncommon in highly endemic areas, with pregnancy and previous surgery to the hepatobiliary tree predisposing to the latter. Nutritional disorders and stunting of growth may occur in children with a moderate to heavy worm burden. Pulmonary ascariasis (eosinophilic or seasonal pneumonitis or Loeffler's syndrome) may occur 4–16 days after infection and presents as a self-limiting pneumonia (cough, dyspnoea and haemoptysis) that resolves in a few weeks.

DIAGNOSIS

- Worms are sometimes passed in the stool or through the mouth or nose, and can be identified macroscopically.
- Finding eggs on faecal microscopy. The best method is examination of a wet mount after concentration using the ethyl sedimentation

technique (see Plates 44, 45). For quantitative assessments of infection, various methods such as the Kato-Katz smear can be used.

- Larvae can be identified in sputum or gastric aspirates during the pulmonary migration phase (examine formalin-fixed organisms for morphology).
- Peripheral eosinophilia may be present (often > 20% of WCC in pulmonary ascariasis).
- In pulmonary ascariasis, CXR shows diffuse pulmonary infiltrates.

TREATMENT

    Mebendazole* ≤ 10 kg: 50 mg twice daily po for 3 days
                 > 10 kg: 100 mg twice daily po for 3 days

or **Albendazole*** ≤ 10 kg: 200 mg single dose po
                 > 10 kg: 400 mg single dose po

or **Pyrantel embonate** 20 mg/kg stat (max. 750 mg) po. Repeat after 1 week if infection heavy. Adverse reactions are common.

---

* Mebendazole and albendazole are not used in pregnancy or in children younger than 6 months.

Intestinal obstruction usually resolves with intravenous fluids, nasogastric suction and specific antihelminthics. **Piperazine citrate** is indicated for both intestinal and biliary obstruction as the narcotising effect on the worm facilitates expulsion.[17,18]

Occasionally **laparotomy** is required.

Corticosteroids are occasionally required in pulmonary ascariasis.

FOLLOW UP

Faecal examination 2–4 weeks post-therapy. Re-treat if eggs are still present.

DRUG AVAILABILITY IN AUSTRALIA

Albendazole   *Eskazole:* 400 mg tabs
                Zentel: 200 mg tabs
Mebendazole   *Banworm:* 100 mg tabs
                Sqworm: 100 mg tabs
                Vermox: 100 mg tabs; 100 mg/5 mL suspension
Piperazine citrate [SAS approval]
Pyrantel embonate   *Anthel:* 125 mg, 250 mg tabs
                     Combantrin: 125 mg, 250 mg tabs
                     Early Bird: 100 mg chocolate squares

Babesia microti

Malaria-like protozoan found in blood

LIFE CYCLE AND EPIDEMIOLOGY

Babesiasis is a zoonosis in which *Babesia microti* is usually transmitted to humans from rodents, cattle or wild animals by the bite of a hard-bodied or ixodid tick (*Ixodes scapularis* is also one of the vectors for *Borrelia burgdorferi*, which causes Lyme disease). The parasites then invade erythrocytes directly (without the exo-erythrocytic liver stage required by human malaria parasites), where they undergo successive cycles of multiplication and reinvasion. Infection can also be acquired through transfusion of blood or blood products.

Human cases are mostly from the north-east coastal area of the USA and are due to *B. microti*. Human infection in Europe is rare and usually occurs in splenectomised patients. Other species (such as *B. divergens*) cause human disease rarely. Although *B. bovis* occurs in Australian cattle, human cases do not occur, possibly because of the feeding preferences of the ticks.

CLINICAL NOTES

In the USA, most infections are asymptomatic or mild. The incubation period is 1–6 weeks. The patient presents with fever, chills, myalgia, fatigue, headache and hepatosplenomegaly. Haemolytic anaemia occurs as a result of erythrocyte infection (usually 1–10% of RBC contain parasites).

It is important to exclude intercurrent Lyme disease in areas where transmission of both diseases occurs. (A case of concurrent infection was described in ProMED, 23 June 1998.)

Splenectomised individuals and those with pre-existing medical disease are at risk of more severe illness. In Europe, all reported patients had been previously splenectomised and presented with fulminant febrile haemolytic disease due to *B. divergens*.

DIAGNOSIS

- Examination of T+T blood smears for intra-erythrocytic parasites. These resemble the ring stages of *Plasmodium falciparum*.
- Haemolytic anaemia results in decreased serum haptoglobin and an elevated reticulocyte count. As in malaria, thrombocytopenia and abnormal LFT are common.

- **Serology** An IFA is available at CDC, Atlanta. Patients' titres often rise to more than 1:1024 during the first weeks of illness and decline gradually over 6 months. Specificity is 100% in patients with other tick-borne diseases or persons not exposed to the parasite. Cross-reactions may occur in serum specimens from patients with malaria infections, but generally titres are lower.

TREATMENT

Patients may recover spontaneously. If the disease is serious, give treatment.

> **Clindamycin** 300–600 mg four times daily parenterally or 600 mg three times daily po for 7–10 days

and **Quinine** 650 mg three or four times daily po for 7–10 days.

Exchange transfusion may be required in profoundly ill patients with high parasitaemia.

FOLLOW UP

Monitor the clinical course and parasitaemia. Convalescence may last 1–18 months.

DRUG AVAILABILITY IN AUSTRALIA

Clindamycin *Dalacin C:* 150 mg caps; 600 mg/4 mL ampoules; 75 mg/5 mL syrup
Quinine sulfate *Quinate:* 300 mg tabs

Balantidium coli

Intestinal ciliated protozoan

LIFE CYCLE AND EPIDEMIOLOGY

Balantidium coli is the only ciliate that is pathogenic to humans. The reservoir host is the pig, although many other mammals may be infected. Trophozoites and/or cysts are excreted in the faeces. Cysts can survive outside the mammalian host for many weeks in moist conditions. Humans are infected by ingestion of cysts in contaminated food and water. Following ingestion, excystation occurs in the small intestine, and the trophozoites colonise the large intestine, where they replicate by binary fission. Cysts are formed and then passed in the faeces. Water-borne outbreaks can occur.

There is a higher incidence in people working in abattoirs and piggeries, especially where personal hygiene is low. The prevalence is highest in Papua New Guinea,[19] Central and South America, and Iran.

CLINICAL NOTES

Asymptomatic carriage is common. *Balantidium coli* may also produce a dysenteric syndrome with rectosigmoid ulceration that resembles amoebic colitis, and which is sometimes complicated by secondary bacteraemia. Symptoms may persist for 1–4 weeks and recur intermittently if not treated. This illness may be associated with severe watery diarrhoea with blood and mucus, and occasionally leads to colonic perforation, peritonitis and death. Appendicitis is rare.

DIAGNOSIS

A wet preparation of a faecal concentrate may reveal large, motile, ciliated trophozoites, as well as cysts (50–70 μm in diameter; see Plate 22). In dysentery cases, scrapings from the ulcer margin may reveal trophozoites. *Balantidium coli* is passed intermittently, and so repeated stool specimens should be examined to enhance parasite detection. Collection of specimens into fixative is preferred, as the organism deteriorates rapidly once outside the intestine.

TREATMENT

Tetracycline   500 mg four times daily po for 10 days

or   **Metronidazole**   750 mg three times daily po for 5 days.

Surgery may be required in fulminant disease.

FOLLOW UP

Monitor the clinical course and repeat faecal microscopy.

DRUG AVAILABILITY IN AUSTRALIA

Metronidazole
  Flagyl: 200 mg, 400 mg tabs; 200 mg/5 mL suspension
  Metrogyl: 200 mg, 400 mg tabs; 200 mg/5 mL suspension
Tetracycline *Tetrex:* 250 mg caps

Blastocystis hominis

Intestinal protozoan

LIFE CYCLE AND EPIDEMIOLOGY

Transmission is by ingestion of contaminated food or water. Epidemiological features are not well defined, but, overcrowding, malnutrition and poor personal hygiene are important factors. Travellers to tropical areas, homosexual men and patients with AIDS have all been reported to have a higher incidence of infection.[20–22] There is a worldwide distribution.

CLINICAL NOTES

The clinical significance of *B. hominis* is controversial and recent studies suggest that it is non-pathogenic in most situations. However, it is sometimes the only organism detected in the setting of acute, watery diarrhoea with abdominal pain, cramps and nausea.[20–23] Diagnostic criteria are included here as guidelines for management of the occasional symptomatic patient with no other obvious cause of diarrhoea.

DIAGNOSIS

Examination of faecal samples for cysts (see Plate 23).[20]

Blastocystis hominis **is** considered to be a pathogen if:
- the patient is persistently symptomatic (> 3 days) and *B. hominis* is the only organism isolated and identified in repeated faecal specimens (and other pathogens have been ruled out), *or*
- *B. hominis* is the only organism identified repeatedly from an immunocompromised patient with symptoms.

Blastocystis hominis is **not** considered to be a pathogen if:
- symptoms resolve spontaneously (< 3 days) and *B. hominis* is not found on repeated examination of faeces, *or*
- *B. hominis* is found with other pathogens (e.g. *Entamoeba histolytica*, *Dientamoeba fragilis*) and treatment for these also eradicates *B. hominis, or*
- *B. hominis* is present in faeces in low numbers only.

TREATMENT

Treatment is not warranted in most cases.

If indicated use:

> **Metronidazole** 400–750 mg three times daily po for 7–10 days.

FOLLOW UP

Faecal examination 2–4 weeks after therapy (ideally include a permanent-stained smear).

DRUG AVAILABILITY IN AUSTRALIA

Metronidazole
Flagyl: 200 mg, 400 mg tabs; 200 mg/5 mL suspension
Metrogyl: 200 mg, 400 mg tabs; 200 mg/5 mL suspension

Capillaria philippinensis

Intestinal nematode of freshwater fish and birds

LIFE CYCLE AND EPIDEMIOLOGY

Larvae are present in the intestine of freshwater fish (the intermediate host). Infection in humans (the definitive host) occurs after eating raw infected freshwater fish. After ingestion, larvae mature to adult worms that burrow into the mucosa of the small intestine. The females produce larvae as well as immature eggs. For this reason, *Capillaria* is one of the few helminths that can maintain the parasite burden by autoinfection (i.e. larvae develop into new adults within the intestine).[24] Eggs passed in the stool are then ingested by freshwater fish. Fish-eating migratory birds may act as reservoir hosts.

Epidemics with significant mortality rates have been reported. *Capillaria philippinensis* occurs mainly in rural communities in the Philippines and Thailand and less commonly in Japan, Taiwan, Iran, Columbia and Egypt. Rare cases of human infections with the animal species *C. hepatica* and *C. aerophila* have been reported worldwide. *Capillaria* spp. have been isolated from rodents and other animals in Australia, but no human cases have been reported.

CLINICAL NOTES

Patients present with diarrhoea and mild abdominal pain a few weeks after infection. As the worm burden increases, the diarrhoea and abdominal pain become more severe and are associated with vomiting, dehydration and prostration. If treatment is delayed, malabsorption and weight loss, and sometimes death, ensue.

Hepatic capillariasis (*C. hepatica*) may cause an acute or subacute hepatitis with eosinophilia, which is sometimes complicated by dissemination to other organs. Pulmonary capillariasis (*C. aerophila*) presents with fever, cough, asthma and pneumonia. Both can be fatal.

DIAGNOSIS

- *Capillaria philippinensis:* eggs, larvae and/or adults in the stool, or in intestinal biopsy. The eggs are similar to *Trichuris trichiuria* ('tea tray' appearance).
- *Capillaria hepatica:* adult worms and/or eggs in liver tissue at biopsy or autopsy. (Identification of *C. hepatica* eggs in the stool is

a spurious finding that results from ingestion of the liver from an infected animal.)
- *Capillaria aerophila:* eggs in the stool or in lung biopsy.
- Electrolyte disturbance, protein-losing enteropathy, and fat, mineral and vitamin malabsorption may be present.

TREATMENT

Albendazole   200 mg twice daily po for 10 days

or   **Mebendazole**   200 mg twice daily po for 20 days (or longer, until eggs are absent in repeated faecal samples).

Electrolyte replacement as required.

FOLLOW UP

Multiple faecal examinations for eggs several months after completion of therapy.

DRUG AVAILABILITY IN AUSTRALIA

Albendazole   *Eskazole:* 400 mg tabs
                  Zentel: 200 mg tabs
Mebendazole   *Banworm:* 100 mg tabs
                  Sqworm: 100 mg tabs
                  Vermox: 100 mg tabs; 100 mg/5 mL suspension

Cryptosporidium parvum

Intestinal coccidian protozoan

LIFE CYCLE AND EPIDEMIOLOGY

Transmission is by the faecal–oral route, as a result of direct person-to-person spread or by drinking water (especially contaminated with human or animal faeces). A low dose of oocysts is sufficient to cause infection.[25] Children, immunocompromised hosts (especially AIDS patients) and travellers are at particular risk of infection. Several water-borne outbreaks have been described in Australia (NSW, ACT and Victoria),[26] including an outbreak linked to an indoor swimming pool. In 1993 an estimated 400 000 persons were affected in a water-borne outbreak in the USA.[27–29] Nosocomial transmission has been reported.[30] Animal-to-person (zoonotic) transmission is known to occur from household pets, and laboratory and farm animals.[1] A food-borne outbreak (chicken salad) has also been reported.[31]

CLINICAL NOTES

The severity and duration of diarrhoeal illness depends on the immune status of the patient. Immunocompetent hosts present with mild to moderate watery diarrhoea lasting 1–20 days (average 10 days) and abdominal pain. Fever may be present, but is usually low-grade. Immunocompromised hosts (especially AIDS patients) may have severe, unrelenting diarrhoea and those with low CD4 counts ($< 0.18 \times 10^9$/L) are often unable to clear the infection. Other clinical syndromes, including cholecystitis, hepatitis, pancreatitis and rarely, respiratory illness, may be seen.

DIAGNOSIS

- Faecal microscopy for oocysts is the mainstay of diagnosis. Many laboratories use modified acid-fast staining of faecal concentrates, although immunofluorescence microscopy using commercially available monoclonal antibodies is the most sensitive and specific method (see Plate 6).

> Specifically request *Cryptosporidium*, as the diagnosis may be missed if only eggs or cyst examination is requested.

- Occasionally, identification of the organism in small intestinal biopsy tissue may be necessary to make the diagnosis.

- **Antigen detection** Several commercial EIA tests are available for the detection of cryptosporidial antigens in stool samples. These kits are reported to be more sensitive than conventional microscopic examination (especially acid-fast staining) and show good correlation with immunofluorescence assays.

TREATMENT

Immunocompetent patient:
Symptomatic treatment and rehydration if required.

Immunocompromised patient:
No agents with proven efficacy.

The following drugs have been used with variable success:[17,32,33]

> **Paromomycin** 1 g twice daily or 500 mg four times daily po for 2 weeks, then maintenance 500 mg twice daily indefinitely to prevent relapse

or **Azithromycin** 1200 mg twice po on day 1, then 1200 mg/day for 27 days, then maintenance 500–750 mg daily long term.

The combination of paromomycin and azithromycin has been reported to produce a greater parasiticidal effect than when either agent is used in monotherapy.[34]

> **Octreotide** 50 mg three times daily sc, increasing the dose slowly in 100 mg increments until a response is obtained (max. 500 mg/day). It has a very marginal effect, but may have some use as a palliative agent for refractory diarrhoea.

Spiramycin and hyperimmune bovine colostrum have also been tried with some effect.

FOLLOW UP

Full recovery may take weeks in immunocompetent individuals. Clinical resolution may occur in immunocompromised patients on treatment, but elimination of the organism is unlikely. In these patients, monitor clinical response and perform stool microscopy (modified acid-fast stain or direct fluorescence) during and after therapy.

DRUG AVAILABILITY IN AUSTRALIA

Azithromycin *Zithromax:* 250 mg, 500 mg, 600 mg tabs; powder for oral suspension 200 mg/5 mL
Octreotide *Sandostatin:* 0.05, 0.1 and 0.5 mg/mL ampoules
Paromomycin [SAS approval] *Humatin:* 250 mg caps

Cyclospora cayetanensis

Intestinal coccidian protozoan

Previously named 'blue-green algae' or 'cyanobacterium-like bodies'.

LIFE CYCLE AND EPIDEMIOLOGY

Transmission of infection is via contaminated water (including tap, roof, tank and aquarium water) as well as swimming in lakes, and food. After ingestion, the oocysts excyst in the GIT, freeing the sporozoites. It is thought that the sporozoites then invade the epithelial cells of the small intestine and undergo asexual multiplication (schizogony). Unsporulated oocysts are passed in the stool, and sporulation does not occur until days to weeks after excretion. (Thus, the oocysts are not infective upon excretion and direct faecal–oral transmission cannot occur.) Whether there are animal reservoir hosts, and the mechanisms of contamination of food and water, are still not fully understood.

Cyclosporiasis is seen in migrants and travellers returning from tropical developing countries. All ages are affected. The disease occurs worldwide, but higher rates are reported from Nepal where outbreaks occur in or following the rainy season. In temperate areas, increased numbers of cases are seen in spring and summer. Consumption of imported fresh fruits and other seasonal produce has been implicated in several outbreaks in the USA and Canada.

CLINICAL NOTES

Patients often present with malaise and low-grade fever, followed by watery diarrhoea, which may be associated with fatigue, myalgia, anorexia, nausea, vomiting and weight loss. Remission usually occurs in 3–4 days, but may be followed by relapses over several weeks. The disease is reported to be more common in HIV-infected individuals. It is usually a self-limited illness in immunocompetent and immuno-compromised patients. However, recurrences in 43% of HIV-infected patients were reported in one study and long-term prophylaxis with co-trimoxazole was required.[35] Biliary disease has also been described in those with concurrent HIV infection. The incubation period is 2–11 (average 7) days.

DIAGNOSIS

Faecal microscopy of wet mounts and stained smears (using modified acid-fast or safranin) is currently the best method for diagnosis.

The organisms are 8–10 μm (approximately twice the size of cryptosporidium oocysts (4–6 μm)). *Cyclospora* oocysts can be excreted intermittently and in small numbers, and so three or more specimens at 2 or 3 day intervals may be required. Concentration procedures should also be used to increase sensitivity (see Plate 7).

Specifically request microscopy for *Cyclospora*, as the diagnosis may be missed if only an egg or cyst examination is requested.

TREATMENT

A self-limiting disease, but recent studies suggest antibiotics may be useful, particularly in HIV-infected patients.[33,35,36]

Trimethoprim-sulfamethoxazole

Immunocompetent patient:
160 mg TMP + 800 mg SMX (i.e. 1 DS tablet) twice po for 3–7 days.

Immunocompromised patient (HIV infection):
160 mg TMP + 800 mg SMX (i.e. 1 DS tablet) four times daily po for 10 days, then 3 times/week.

FOLLOW UP

Monitor the clinical course, repeat stool examination.

DRUG AVAILABILITY IN AUSTRALIA

Trimethoprim-sulfamethoxazole
Bactrim or *Septrin* or *Resprim:* 80 mg, 400 mg tabs
Bactrim DS or *Septrin Forte* or *Resprim Forte:* 160 mg, 800 mg tabs

Dientamoeba fragilis

Intestinal amoeba-like protozoan

The epidemiology is not yet well understood although *D. fragilis* infection appears to have a worldwide distribution. Transmission via the faecal–oral route has not been documented. Transmission via helminth eggs, such as *Enterobius* spp., is likely. There is no cyst stage. *Dientamoeba fragilis* is now considered a trichomonad.

CLINICAL NOTES

Pathogenicity is not well defined. The most common symptoms are diarrhoea, abdominal discomfort, nausea, anorexia, poor weight gain and fatigue, particularly in children.

DIAGNOSIS

Demonstration of trophozoites (no cyst form) by faecal microscopy. A permanent-stained smear is necessary, so specimens must be examined immediately or preserved in fixative. It is easy to confuse *D. fragilis* with non-pathogenic organisms (such as *Endolimax nana* and *Entamoeba hartmanni*). The organism has been cultured on Boeck and Drbohlav's medium.[37] This infection is likely to be under-diagnosed because a permanent-stained faecal smear is not performed routinely in many laboratories (see Plate 17).

TREATMENT

Doxycycline   100 mg twice daily for 10 days

or   **Paromomycin**
Children: 25–30 mg/kg per day in 3 doses for 7 days
Adults: 500 mg three times daily po for 7 days

or   **Diiodohydroxyquin**   650 mg three times daily po for 20 days.

Metronidazole is reported as efficacious in some cases.

Also treat concurrent *Enterobius vermicularis* infection if present.

FOLLOW UP

Repeat faecal examination 2–4 weeks after therapy (including a permanent-stained smear).

DRUG AVAILABILITY IN AUSTRALIA

Diiodohydroxyquin or **iodoquinol** *Yodoxin:* not currently available
in Australia
Doxycycline *Doryx:* 50 mg, 100 mg caps
Vibramycin: 50 mg, 100 mg tabs
Paromomycin [SAS approval] *Humatin:* 250 mg caps

Diphyllobothrium latum

Cestode: fish tapeworm

Infection is acquired by eating raw, pickled or inadequately cooked freshwater fish containing infective larvae. The larvae mature to adult worms (which can grow to more than 10 metres) in the small intestine, and egg production commences in about 5 weeks. Immature eggs are passed in faeces and, under appropriate conditions, mature over 11–15 days. Further maturation occurs after ingestion by a freshwater crustacean (copepod, which is the first intermediate host). Following ingestion of the copepod by a suitable freshwater fish (second intermediate host), the larva migrates into the fish flesh where it develops into a plerocercoid larva (sparganum). If the smaller infected fish is eaten by a larger one, the sparganum may migrate into the flesh of the larger fish. Mammals other than humans can also be infected.

Infection is endemic in Europe (especially the Baltic countries), Siberia, Japan, North America, Uganda and Chile. Individuals from Finland are genetically predisposed to anaemia. The domestic dog may act as a reservoir host.

CLINICAL NOTES

Diphyllobothriasis is usually asymptomatic, but this depends on the number of worms. Symptoms may include abdominal discomfort, diarrhoea, vomiting and weight loss. Infection may be complicated by intestinal obstruction and/or megaloblastic anaemia due to vitamin B12 deficiency (or, rarely, folate deficiency). Worms may survive for 30 years, and so infection may be long lasting. Migration of proglottids can cause cholecystitis or cholangitis.

DIAGNOSIS

- Demonstration of eggs and, occasionally, characteristic proglottids with a central uterus, by microscopic examination of faeces (see Plate 33).
- Peripheral eosinophilia with slight leucocytosis may occur.

TREATMENT

Praziquantel* 2.5–10 mg/kg stat po for adults and children over 4 years of age (*Caution in lactating mothers)

or **Niclosamide** Children 11–34 kg: 1 g stat po
                                              > 34 kg: 1.5 g stat po
                         Adults   2 g stat po

Patients may benefit from nutritional replacement therapy. Vitamin B12 deficiency should be treated parenterally.

FOLLOW UP

Faecal examination for eggs and proglottids at 1 and 3 months after therapy.

DRUG AVAILABILITY IN AUSTRALIA

Niclosamide *Yomesan:* not currently available in Australia
Praziquantel *Biltricide:* 600 mg tabs

Dirofilaria immitis

Filarial nematode: dog heartworm

LIFE CYCLE AND EPIDEMIOLOGY

This common zoonotic filarial infection is found mainly in dogs and also in other wild animals, including kangaroos in Australia. Forty species are reported worldwide, but only *D. immitis* has been reported as a pathogen in humans. Microfilariae are present in the dog's blood and the adult worms are found in the right ventricle of the heart. Adult worms are very long (female 25–30 cm; males 12–18 cm). Transmission is by mosquito bite. In humans the worms do not reach maturity and no microfilariae can be detected.

The infection occurs in tropical, subtropical and warm temperate regions of the world. In Australia, the prevalence is very high in dogs in Northern Queensland,[38] but the disease is enzootic as far south as Melbourne.

CLINICAL NOTES

Many patients are asymptomatic. In symptomatic patients, pulmonary lesions are most common and may present with haemoptysis. The lesions are mainly peripheral and sharply defined on imaging (coin lesions). It is important to exclude malignancy. Dead or dying worms may be found in the lesions. Many cases are diagnosed post-mortem. Sometimes patients present with infections in the skin, peritoneal cavity, ocular tissue and other sites,[38] which usually have a benign course, but may present with pain, swelling and pruritis, especially when the eye is involved.

DIAGNOSIS

- The diagnosis rests on identification of the worm in biopsy material from the lesion. The worm is often difficult to recognise in tissue sections because of the chronic nature of the infection and the probability that the worm will have been absorbed by the time the tissue is looked at (usually post-mortem). Routine histology is useful if the infection is current and the worm is still alive. Knowledge of nematode anatomy is essential to identify the worm in section.

Unlike other filarial nematodes, microfilariae
are **not** found in blood or tissue in human cases.

- Moderate eosinophilia may be present.
- Serology is not useful because of low sensitivity and specificity.

TREATMENT

Surgical removal of the worm if the infection is localised to a subcutaneous or ocular site.

Medical therapy is not usually required.

FOLLOW UP

Monitor the clinical course.

Dracunculus medinensis

Tissue nematode: guinea worm

Humans acquire infection by drinking unfiltered water (usually from 'step' wells) containing copepods ('water fleas') infected with *D. medinensis*. Following ingestion, the released larvae penetrate the duodenal wall and develop in loose connective tissue in the abdominal cavity and retroperitoneal space. The female worms then migrate through the deep connective tissue to the dermis. Approximately one year after infection, the female worm induces a blister on the skin that ruptures. When this lesion comes into contact with water, the female worm emerges and releases larvae into the water. Larvae can then be ingested by a copepod.

Infection is endemic in Africa and, until recently, in the Middle East and India. In developed countries, guinea worm is occasionally diagnosed in a returned traveller or in a migrant from an endemic area.

In endemic countries, this infection has serious economic consequences because a substantial proportion of the population is incapacitated for weeks each year. A successful WHO global eradication program has reduced the number of cases dramatically (by 97%).[39] Yemen and 16 African countries are yet to be declared free of dracunculosis.[40]

CLINICAL NOTES

The blister is usually found on the lower extremities. It develops into a red papule just before rupture, and larvae are discharged into the water as the worm protrudes through the ulcer. Patients may have a generalised reaction, with urticaria, vomiting, diarrhoea and dyspnoea, at the time of blister formation. Symptoms improve when the larvae and worm metabolites are discharged. If the worm is incompletely removed an inflammatory response occurs (and frequently also secondary bacterial infection) and the patient may be bedridden for many weeks.

DIAGNOSIS

• Usually diagnosed clinically, but larvae may be demonstrated in the fluid from the blister (this may be enhanced by immersing the affected part in water).

- Morphological identification of the adult worm may be possible after its removal from the blister.
- The calcified worms may be apparent on X-rays.

TREATMENT

Local cleansing of the lesion and local application of antibiotics followed by physical removal of the worm over several days by slowly winding it onto a stick or rod.

Drugs have little effect on the worm or larvae, but may decrease inflammation and facilitate removal of the worm.

Metronidazole
Children: 25 mg/kg per day (max. 750 mg/day) three times daily for 10 days
Adults: 250 mg three times daily for 10 days

or **Thiabendazole** 25–37.5 mg/kg twice daily for 3 days.

FOLLOW UP

Monitor the clinical course; radiological examination for calcified worms.

DRUG AVAILABILITY IN AUSTRALIA

Metronidazole
Flagyl: 200 mg, 400 mg tabs; 200 mg/5 mL suspension
Metrogyl: 200 mg, 400 mg tabs; 200 mg/5 mL suspension
Thiabendazole *Mintezol:* 500 mg tabs

Echinococcus spp.

Cestodes: canine tapeworms

Echinococcus granulosus (cystic hydatid disease)

LIFE CYCLE AND EPIDEMIOLOGY

Dogs or other canines (definitive host) harbour the adult hydatid tapeworm. Eggs are released and passed in the faeces. After ingestion by an intermediate host (usually sheep, goats, pigs, cattle and horses, but also humans), the eggs hatch in the small bowel and release oncospheres that penetrate the intestinal wall and migrate via the circulatory system to various organs, especially the liver and lungs. In these organs, the oncosphere develops into a gradually enlarging cyst that produces protoscolices and daughter cysts that fill the cyst interior. Dogs become infected by ingesting the cyst-containing organs of the infected intermediate host.

A cycle involving wild animals, including kangaroos, feral pigs, dingoes and domestic dogs that live on the outskirts of cities, also exists.[41,42]

There is a worldwide distribution. Cases are still reported from south-eastern and north-western Australia; a recent study detected 195 new cases in NSW and the ACT during a 5-year period.[43]

CLINICAL NOTES

Cysts may occur in the liver (50–70%), lungs (20–30%) and elsewhere (brain, heart, bones muscle etc. < 10%). However, infections may be asymptomatic for years. Symptoms depend on the size and site of the expanding cyst. Liver cysts may cause abdominal discomfort and, rarely, biliary tract obstruction. Pulmonary involvement can produce chest pain, cough and haemoptysis. Complications occur in less than 10% of cases and include secondary bacterial infection, cyst leakage or rupture with allergic manifestations (fever, urticaria, eosinophilia, anaphylaxis), and/or dissemination of daughter cysts. In rare cases, there may be direct vascular invasion.

DIAGNOSIS

- Radiological imaging with CT or ultrasound is the mainstay of diagnosis.
- **Serology** Most laboratories in Australia use the IHA as a screening test. The sensitivity of this test is approximately 88% in

patients with hydatid liver cysts, but cross-reactions with *Taenia solium* occur. Hydatid cysts in the lung, and dead or calcified cysts, are less frequently associated with positive serology (25–56%) than are active cysts in the liver. Low titres (64–128) have been observed with collagen diseases, liver cirrhosis, schistosomiasis and other parasitic infections. An EIA is thought to have similar sensitivity and specificity as the IHA.[44] The Arc 5 IEP test is used as a confirmatory test and also to monitor patients after treatment.

- The surgically removed cyst or cyst fluid removed under radiological guidance may be examined for scolices (or hooklets) although diagnostic aspiration is not recommended because of the risk of dissemination (see Plates 28–31).
- Eosinophilia is present in 20–25% of patients.

TREATMENT

Surgical removal of operable cysts is still the treatment of choice. Chemotherapy with albendazole should be considered prior to surgery. Particular care is required during surgery to avoid spillage of cyst contents, as this is a major predictor for recurrent disease.

PAIR therapy has been shown to be effective for treating uncomplicated hepatic cysts in small numbers of patients. 'PAIR' stands for **P**uncture; **A**spiration of cyst contents (using a fine needle or catheter under CT guidance); **I**ntroduction of a scolicidal agent (e.g. alcohol or hypertonic saline); and **R**e-aspiration of the solution. It is recommended that patients receive medical therapy for 2 months before the procedure. Endoscopic retrograde cholangiopancreatography (ERCP) should be performed before surgery to rule out possible connections of the cyst with the biliary tree.[45]

> **Albendazole** Two to four cycles of 400 mg twice daily po for 28 days are given with a 2-week rest period between cycles. (The rest period was originally recommended for safety reasons. However, continuous therapy does not seem to be related to increased risk from side effects.)

Chemotherapy alone should be reserved for use in patients with inoperable disease or after incomplete surgery (WHO recommendation). Preoperative therapy decreases larval viability, and postoperative therapy appears to reduce the risk of recurrences. Guidelines for the duration of perioperative chemotherapy are lacking, but a reasonable approach would be to treat for 2 months before, and in some cases 2–4 weeks after surgery. WCC and LFT should be monitored fortnightly while on therapy. If chemotherapy is used alone, an efficacy of 50–77% is reported. The best results have been obtained when medical therapy is used as an adjunct to surgery or to PAIR.

In refractory cases **combination therapy** with albendazole and praziquantel as well as **repeated surgery** may be required.

FOLLOW UP

Monitor the clinical response to therapy by imaging (look for a reduction in size and a change in consistency of the cyst). The Arc 5 IEP test is also useful for monitoring the decreasing antibody levels after successful surgical and/or medical therapy. Repeat the test 3–6 months after therapy.

Echinococcus multilocularis (alveolar hydatid disease)

LIFE CYCLE AND EPIDEMIOLOGY

Echinococcus multilocularis is transmitted by wild canines (usually red or arctic foxes). Small rodents are the main intermediate hosts, and humans are infected accidentally. Larval growth (in the liver) remains indefinitely in the proliferative stage, resulting in invasion of the surrounding tissues.

Echinococcus multilocularis occurs in the Northern hemisphere in Europe, Asia, North America, and has also been reported from South America. The overall prevalence is unknown, but one study recorded a seroprevalence of 8.8% in China.[46]

Echinococcus vogeli (polycystic hydatid disease) is reported from areas of Central and South America and is transmitted by the bush dog, and occasionally domestic dogs, with pacas, rats and possums acting as the intermediate hosts. Human disease is rare.

CLINICAL NOTES

The liver is involved in 92–100% of cases and, unlike the hydatid cysts of *E. granulosus*, *E. multilocularis* presents as an expansive and infiltrative tumour that may be mistaken for a malignancy. Invasion of adjacent structures and distant metastases to the lungs and brain can occur. Abdominal pain, hepatomegaly and jaundice are the commonest presenting features.

Echinococcus vogeli affects mainly the liver, where it acts as a slow-growing tumor.

DIAGNOSIS

- Radiological imaging, especially CT and ultrasound, shows an irregular hepatic lesion with microcalcifications.

- **Serology** Tests for *E. granulosus* also detect antibodies to *E. multilocularis*. Recently tests have been developed using specific antigen fractions of *E. multilocularis* that distinguish between the two infections.

TREATMENT

Radical surgery remains the treatment of choice.

Albendazole has been shown to have some activity in animal models and limited human studies and should be considered as an adjunct to surgery or in inoperable cases: 400 mg twice daily in cycles for many months (may be required for years).

FOLLOW UP

Monitor with regular imaging and serology as for *E. granulosus*.

DRUG AVAILABILITY IN AUSTRALIA

Albendazole *Eskazole:* 400 mg tabs
                 Zentel: 200 mg tabs
Praziquantel *Biltricide:* 600 mg tabs

Entamoeba histolytica

Intestinal protozoan: commonly called amoeba

Among parasites amoebiasis is the third leading cause of death after malaria and schistosomiasis. Transmission is mostly via the faecal–oral route (often due to preparation of food by infected individuals). Excystation occurs in the small intestine and trophozoites then migrate to the large intestine. The trophozoites multiply by binary fission and produce cysts, which are passed in formed stools. The cysts can survive days to weeks in the environment and are responsible for transmission. Trophozoites may invade the intestinal mucosa or, through the bloodstream, extra-intestinal sites such as the liver, brain and lungs, and cause extra-intestinal amoebiasis.

There is a high prevalence in developing countries, although the infection occurs worldwide. Those at most risk in developed countries are returned travellers, migrants from developing countries and male homosexuals.[47] The high prevalence in homosexual men is predominantly due to an increase in infections with a non-pathogenic species, *Entamoeba dispar*.

Intestinal amoebiasis Asymptomatic cyst carriage of pathogenic and non-pathogenic strains occurs. Non-invasive infection (i.e. serum antibody negative) with presumed pathogenic stains may cause mild gastrointestinal symptoms.

Invasive intestinal disease has a gradual onset of abdominal pain, loose stools or diarrhoea. All patients have haem-positive stools. In severe cases there is dysentery and fever, occasionally complicated by fulminant colitis, appendicitis and/or toxic megacolon. Chronic amoebic colitis may be misdiagnosed as inflammatory bowel disease. Colonic amoeboma may mimic colonic carcinoma.

Extra-intestinal amoebiasis Liver abscesses usually present with abrupt onset of abdominal pain and fever associated with marked hepatic tenderness; 20–40% of patients have diarrhoea. Most travellers present within 2–5 months of leaving a high prevalence area. Cyst extension or rupture may involve the pleural space and lung parenchyma, pericardium or peritoneal cavity. Brain abscess, and cutaneous and genital amoebic lesions, are rare. There may be PUO.

DIAGNOSIS

- Microscopic examination of faecal specimens for trophozoites and cysts (look for erythrophagocytic trophozoites as an indicator of invasiveness). Specimens may include dysenteric stool specimens, sigmoidoscopy/colonoscopy fluid or biopsy tissue. Microscopy is seldom positive in extra-intestinal amoebiasis.

Entamoeba dispar is morphologically identical to *E. histolytica* and is differentiated on the basis of isoenzymatic, immunological or molecular analysis.

Entamoeba coli and *E. hartmanni* are differentiated from *E. histolytica* on the basis of the morphological characteristics of the cysts and trophozoites. (See Plates 12–16.)

- An EIA for antigen detection in faeces is now widely available and can distinguish *E. histolytica* from *E. dispar.* This test is performed at VIDRL and ICPMR.
- The diagnosis of extra-intestinal amoebiasis is based on clinical and epidemiological features and the early use of non-invasive imaging studies (such as CT scanning and ultrasound) of an abscess.
- Leucocytosis and elevated ESR occur in 80–90%, and abnormal LFT in 72%, of patients with amoebic liver abscess. These tests are usually normal in intestinal amoebiasis.
- **Serology** An IHA is commonly available and is the investigation of choice in extra-intestinal amoebiasis. It has a specificity of 98% and a sensitivity for extra-intestinal disease of 91–95%, 84% for invasive intestinal disease and 9% for asymptomatic carriers.

  IHA antibody titres remain elevated for years after the invasive disease has been successfully treated. An EIA, which appears to be more sensitive and specific than the IHA, is also available. Results become negative 6–12 months after effective treatment.
- Microscopy of aspirated material from the wall (not the central necrotic material) of rectal ulcers or a liver abscess may reveal trophozoites, although this procedure is not commonly performed.

TREATMENT

Cyst passers:

Diloxanide furoate 500 mg three times daily po for 10 days

or **Paromomycin** 500 mg three times daily po for 7 days.

Invasive rectocolitis:

Metronidazole   750–800 mg three times daily po for 6–10 days

or   **Tinidazole**   2 g once daily po for 2–3 days (up to 10 days)

and **Diloxanide furoate**   500 mg three times daily po for 10 days.

Liver abscess:

Metronidazole   750–800 mg three times daily iv or po for 14 days

or   **Tinidazole**   2 g once daily po for 5 days

and **Diloxanide furoate**   500 mg three times daily po for 10 days.

Needle aspiration of the abscess should be considered, depending on the risk of rupture (i.e. abscess > 6 cm, location near to the pericardium or the liver surface or in the left lobe of the liver) and whether there has been a response to medical therapy in 3–5 days.

Surgery should be reserved for those with a ruptured abscess, bacterial superinfection or when the abscess is inaccessible for needle aspiration.

FOLLOW UP

Intestinal:
Faecal examination 2–4 weeks after therapy and careful clinical follow up to rule out extra-intestinal disease.

Extra-intestinal:
Monitor the clinical response to therapy and the size of the abscess with ultrasound. It may take months for abscesses to disappear after successful treatment.

DRUG AVAILABILITY IN AUSTRALIA

Diloxanide furoate [SAS approval]   *Furamide:* 500 mg tabs (Contact Boots for direct importation.)
Metronidazole
   Flagyl: 200 mg, 400 mg tabs; 200 mg/5 mL suspension
   Metrogyl: 200 mg, 400 mg tabs; 200 mg/5 mL suspension
Paromomycin [SAS approval]   *Humatin:* 250 mg caps
Tinidazole   *Fasigyn:* 500 mg tabs
      Simplotan: 500 mg tabs

Enterobius vermicularis

Intestinal nematode: also called pin worm or threadworm

LIFE CYCLE AND EPIDEMIOLOGY

Infection is acquired by ingesting eggs, usually from contaminated hands, but also from food and less commonly water. Larvae pass from the small to the large intestine where they become mature. After approximately 1 month, gravid females migrate nocturnally and deposit eggs on the perianal or perineal skin. The larvae mature inside the eggs and the eggs become infectious within 6 hours. Eggs stuck under fingernails during scratching are the commonest source of infection. Person-to-person transmission can also occur by handling contaminated clothes or bed linen. The life span of the adult worms is about 2 months.

There is a worldwide distribution, with infections occurring more commonly among children aged 5–10 years, especially in schools and within family groups.

CLINICAL NOTES

The infection is often asymptomatic. The most common symptom is nocturnal anal pruritus. Occasionally migration of the adult worm has been implicated in appendicitis and chronic salpingitis.

DIAGNOSIS

- Microscopic identification of eggs collected in the perianal area is the best method for diagnosing enterobiasis. A perineal 'sticky tape' preparation ('Scotch-tape' or 'Sellotape' test) is collected early in the morning before bathing or defaecation. This is then transferred to a slide for examination for worms and eggs. An anal swab may also be used. Eggs are occasionally found in the stool (see Plate 48).
- Eosinophilia may be present.

TREATMENT

Mebendazole
Children: 100 mg stat po, repeat after 2 weeks
Adults: 100–200 mg stat po, repeat after 2 weeks

or **Albendazole** 400 mg stat, repeat after 2 weeks, is also effective

or   **Pyrantel embonate** (less commonly used because of frequent
side effects)
Children: 20 mg/kg stat (max. 750 mg), repeat after 2 weeks
Adults: 20 mg/kg stat (max. 750 mg), repeat after 2 weeks

> Drug treatment is recommended for all family members, as
> well as thorough washing of family bed linen.

FOLLOW UP

Monitor the clinical response. Follow up with another 'Scotch-tape'
test if symptoms persist (it may take 4–6 consecutive negative tapes
to rule out infection).

DRUG AVAILABILITY IN AUSTRALIA

Albendazole   *Eskazole:* 400 mg tabs
                  Zentel: 200 mg tabs
Mebendazole   *Banworm:* 100 mg tabs
                  Sqworm: 100 mg tabs
                  Vermox: 100 mg tabs; 100 mg/5 mL suspension
Pyrantel embonate   *Anthel:* 125 mg, 250 mg tabs
                        Combantrin: 125 mg, 250 mg tabs
                        Early Bird: 100 mg chocolate squares

Fasciola gigantica, Fasciola hepatica

Trematodes: cattle/sheep liver flukes

LIFE CYCLE AND EPIDEMIOLOGY

Mammals acquire infection by ingestion of the infective stage (metacercariae) on uncooked aquatic plants such as watercress. The metacercariae penetrate the intestinal wall and then the hepatic capsule and parenchyma to reach their final destination, the large biliary ducts. The long-lived adult flukes reside in the biliary tracts of sheep, goats and cattle, and humans are accidental hosts. Immature eggs are passed in the stool and, after development in water, miracidia are released and invade the intermediate host (snails). Cercariae are released from the snail and encyst on water vegetation. Maturation from metacercariae into adult flukes takes 3–4 months in humans.

Fasciola hepatica has a worldwide distribution including Australia[48] whereas *F. gigantica*, which mainly infects cattle, is more commonly found in South East Asia and Africa. Both are most common where livestock are intensively farmed and where humans consume raw watercress.

CLINICAL NOTES

Most human infections are mild. During the early migratory phase (2 months after infection) there may be epigastric or RUQ abdominal pain, fever, hepatomegaly, vomiting, diarrhoea, urticaria and eosinophilia (up to 80% of WCC).

When the flukes enter the bile canaliculi approximately 3 weeks later (or sometimes longer), these symptoms subside. In the chronic phase, cholangitis and cholecystitis may result from adult flukes in the bile ducts. Bile duct obstruction and biliary cirrhosis are rare. Ectopic migration to skin, lung and brain occurs and may result in nodules or abscesses.

DIAGNOSIS

- The diagnosis is made in the chronic stage by microscopic examination of multiple faecal or bile samples for *F. hepatica* eggs. Formalin-ether concentration is desirable. The eggs are very similar to those of *Fasciolopsis buski*. Pseudofascioliasis refers to the presence of eggs in the stool resulting from recent ingestion of infected livers containing eggs.

- **Serology** An EIA using soluble antigen from adult flukes detects circulating antibodies. Serodiagnosis is important in the indirect diagnosis of acute fascioliasis because eggs may not be detected for up to 12 weeks, and also for chronic fascioliasis when egg production may be low or intermittent. It is also useful to rule out pseudofascioliasis. Antibody levels may remain elevated for years, even after successful treatment. Cross-reactivity has been reported with sera from patients with schistosomiasis.
- CT, ultrasound or cholangiography may show hepatic and biliary abnormalities.

TREATMENT

Triclabendazole 12 mg/kg once daily po for 1–2 days.[49,50]

Use **corticosteroids** and **antibiotics** to dampen the inflammatory response to the flukes and to treat secondary bacterial infection.

> Praziquantel is **not** effective. Bithionol is used in some countries, but its efficacy is questionable (cure rate ≈ 50%).

DRUG AVAILABILITY IN AUSTRALIA

Triclabendazole [SAS approval] *Fasinex®* 12% suspension
(may be obtained from Ciba-Geigy Laboratories, Basel, Switzerland)

Fasciolopsis buski and *Brachylaima* spp.

Trematodes: intestinal flukes

Humans acquire infection by ingesting uncooked aquatic plants (water chestnuts, bamboo shoots etc.) on which the organisms have encysted. The infective form (metacercariae) can survive in the environment for up to 1 year. After ingestion, mature worms develop in the duodenum and jejunum within 3 months. Eggs are excreted and, on reaching fresh water, the larvae hatch and invade intermediate hosts (specific snails) in which further maturation takes place, before free-swimming cercariae emerge and attach and encyst on various water plants. *Fasciolopsis buski* reservoir hosts include pigs, dogs and rabbits; it is mainly found in Asian countries, especially Thailand, Malaysia, Indonesia, India, Bangladesh, Myanmar and southern China, in areas where humans raise pigs and consume freshwater plants.

Unrelated intestinal flukes, *Brachylaima* spp., have been discovered in South Australia where children acquired infection by ingestion of infected snails.[51]

CLINICAL NOTES

Most infections are asymptomatic. Abdominal pain, nausea, vomiting and diarrhoea may occur in heavier infections. Intestinal obstruction, malabsorption, peripheral oedema and ascites may develop in the most severe cases.

DIAGNOSIS

- Microscopic demonstration of large operculated eggs (130×80 μm) in faeces or vomitus. The eggs are very similar to those of *Fasciola hepatica*.
- Leucocytosis and eosinophilia may be present.

TREATMENT

	Praziquantel	75 mg/kg per day po in 3 doses over 1 or 2 days
or	**Niclosamide**	2 g single dose, chewed (cheaper, but less effective).

FOLLOW UP

Faecal examinations for eggs at 1 month after therapy.

DRUG AVAILABILITY IN AUSTRALIA

Niclosamide *Yomesan:* not currently available in Australia
Praziquantel *Biltricide:* 600 mg tabs

Giardia duodenalis

Intestinal flagellate protozoan,
also known as *G. lamblia* and *G. intestinalis*

LIFE CYCLE AND EPIDEMIOLOGY

Infection is acquired by ingestion of cysts in contaminated food and water, or through person-to-person contact. Excystation occurs in the small intestine and the trophozoite is responsible for producing gastrointestinal symptoms. Encystation occurs as the parasites pass towards the colon, and cysts are found in normal (non-diarrhoeal) faeces. The cysts can survive several months in cold water. Travel, infancy and young childhood, particularly if attending a childcare centre, immunodeficiency and an active homosexual life style are risk factors. There is evidence that giardiasis is a zoonosis and that animals contribute to contamination of surface water. There is a worldwide distribution.

CLINICAL NOTES

Infection may be asymptomatic or present as acute self-limiting diarrhoea with epigastric pain, nausea, bloating and flatulence. Steatorrhoea and weight loss are common. The incubation period is 1–2 weeks. Most patients have had diarrhoea for 1–2 weeks on presentation and, if untreated, symptoms resolve in 1–2 months.

Chronic symptoms, which include intermittent diarrhoea, malabsorption, weight loss and malaise, occur in 30–50% of patients and may go on for months. Post-giardiasis lactose intolerance may persist for weeks after treatment. In children nutritional insufficiency can retard growth and development.

DIAGNOSIS

- The passage of organisms in the stool may be intermittent, and so repeated microscopic examination of multiple faecal specimens for trophozoites or cysts (using wet preparations and permanent smears) may be required to confirm the diagnosis. The formalin-ether concentration technique may not be as effective as expected for *G. duodenalis*. The organism is detected in more than 90% of cases if these techniques are applied carefully (see Plates 18–21).

- An Entero-Test capsule or gastroscopy may be required to collect duodenal contents and/or tissue for examination for trophozoites in difficult cases.
- EIA for antigen detection in faeces and immunofluorescence for detection of parasites are both available as commercial kits.

TREATMENT

Metronidazole*
Children: 15 mg/kg per day in 3 doses for 3–7 days
Adults: 2 g (single dose) for 3 days (efficacy >90%)
or 400 mg three times daily for 3–7 days

or **Tinidazole**
Children: 50–75 mg/kg per day (single dose)
Adults: 2 g stat po (efficacy >90%).

Albendazole is also effective.[17]

If necessary, treat pregnant women in the first trimester with:

Paromomycin 25–30 mg/kg per day in 3 doses for 5–10 days.[33] *Limited information available, but no reports of congenital abnormalities.*

---

* Metronidazole is considered safe in the second and third trimesters of pregnancy, but should be avoided in the first trimester.

FOLLOW UP

Faecal examinations two weeks to one month post-therapy should be performed to verify parasite clearance (include a permanent-stained smear). An Entero-Test or gastroscopy and duodenal aspirate or biopsy may be required if stools are negative and the patient continues to have symptoms.

DRUG AVAILABILITY IN AUSTRALIA

Metronidazole
Flagyl: 200 mg, 400 mg tabs; 200 mg/5 mL suspension
Metrogyl: 200 mg, 400 mg tabs; 200 mg/5 mL suspension
Paromomycin **[SAS approval]** *Humatin:* 250 mg caps
Tinidazole *Fasigyn:* 500 mg tabs
Simplotan: 500 mg tabs

Gnathostoma spinigerum

Tissue nematode

In wild and domestic felines and canines (the definitive hosts), the adult worms reside in the gastric wall. Eggs are passed in the faeces and, after maturation in water, the larvae are ingested by small crustacea (first intermediate host). Fish, frogs or snakes ingest the crustacea (second intermediate host) and the larvae further mature in their flesh. These animals may be ingested by the definitive host or by other animals (paratenic hosts). In the latter case, the larvae do not develop further, but remain infective for the next predator. Human gnathostomiasis is acquired by the ingestion of infected, undercooked fish, shrimps, crayfish, crabs, chicken, ducks and other birds, pork, frogs and snakes, and also by drinking water containing infected crustacea. In humans, the larvae do not mature completely and cause pathology by wandering around the body.

The infection is endemic in South East Asia and is most common in Thailand. It is also prevalent in Japan, China and the Philippines.

CLINICAL NOTES

Nausea and vomiting may coincide with penetration of the intestinal wall by the immature worms. Later, migration in the subcutaneous tissue causes migratory swellings that are similar to CLM. These are often associated with pruritis, erythema and pain. Each swelling is hard and non-pitting and may last for weeks. Migration in other tissues can result in cough, haematuria and ocular (iris holes, uveitis and subretinal haemorrhage) and neurological involvement. If untreated, the parasite may migrate through the spinal cord, causing a painful radiculomyelopathy with intense girdle pain and paraparesis, and then into the brain. Death may result from brain stem involvement. *Gnathostoma spinigerum* is therefore a cause of eosinophilic meningitis and myeloencephalitis.

DIAGNOSIS

- Confirmed by removal and identification of larvae.
- Serology is not routinely available in Australia.
- Marked eosinophilia in blood and/or CSF (35–80%) may be present.

TREATMENT

Surgical removal of the larvae is the most effective therapy, if possible.

Medical therapy may be used as an alternative where surgery is not possible.

  Albendazole 400–800 mg twice daily po for 21 days

or **Mebendazole** 200 mg po every 3 hours for 6 days.

Corticosteroids are used in the management of eosinophilic meningitis.

FOLLOW UP

Monitor the clinical course and eosinophilia, and use serology (if available).

DRUG AVAILABILITY IN AUSTRALIA

Albendazole *Eskazole:* 400 mg tabs
      Zentel: 200 mg tabs
Mebendazole *Banworm:* 100 mg tabs
      Sqworm: 100 mg tabs
      Vermox: 100 mg tabs; 100 mg/5 mL suspension

Hookworms

Intestinal nematodes

Ancylostoma duodenale (Old World hookworm)

Necator americanus (New World hookworm)

LIFE CYCLE AND EPIDEMIOLOGY

The two species of human hookworms are very similar. Larvae penetrate through intact skin, especially the feet, in areas where shoes are not worn (*A. duodenale* can also be transmitted via the oral route). Larvae are carried to the pulmonary capillaries where they migrate into the lungs, penetrate the pulmonary alveoli, ascend the bronchial tree to the pharynx, and are swallowed. Adult worms live in the lumen of the small intestine attached to the mucosa, which causes chronic blood loss. After about 5 weeks, eggs are passed in the stool and, under favourable conditions (moisture, warmth and shade), hatch in 1–2 days. Larvae are released, grow in the faeces or the soil, and after 5–10 days become filariform larvae that are infective and can survive 3–4 weeks in favourable environments. Adult worms have a life span of 1–2 years.

Hookworm infection is found mostly in poor and rural communities worldwide, especially where there is faecal contamination of the soil and high humidity. The two species have overlapping geographic distributions. *Ancylostoma duodenale* now appears to be the predominant species in Australia, and is endemic amongst Aboriginal communities in northern Western Australia and the Northern Territory.[52,53]

CLINICAL NOTES

Some patients (especially non-immune expatriates or travellers) develop a pruritic rash or 'ground itch' at the larval penetration site. Migration of larvae through the lungs may produce cough, wheeze, fever and eosinophilia within 1–2 weeks of infection. This phase is self-limiting, lasting 1–2 months. As the adult worms attach to the intestinal mucosa, epigastric pain, nausea, vomiting, diarrhoea and weight loss may occur. Iron deficiency anaemia and chronic malnutrition are the major problems in chronic infections, especially in children (with *A. duodenale*, the blood loss is of the order of 0.1 mL/worm per day).

DIAGNOSIS

- Microscopic demonstration of eggs in the faeces. Concentration methods are necessary to detect light infections, and hookworm eggs need to be differentiated from *Trichostrongylus* eggs. For quantitative assessments of infection, various methods, such as a Kato-Katz smear, can be used. Examination of the eggs does not distinguish between *N. americanus* and *A. duodenale*. However, Harada culture of a faecal specimen may produce filariform larvae, which can be used to differentiate between hookworms and *Strongyloides stercoralis* (see Plates 51–54).
- Peripheral eosinophilia may be present.

TREATMENT

Mebendazole*
≤ 10 kg : 50 mg twice daily po for 3 days
> 10 kg : 100 mg twice daily po for 3 days

or **Albendazole***
≤ 10 kg : 200 mg single dose po
> 10 kg : 400 mg single dose po

---
* Mebendazole and albendazole are **not** used in pregnancy
or in children younger than 6 months.
---

or **Pyrantel embonate** 20 mg/kg stat po (max. 750 mg). Repeat after 1 week if infestation heavy.

Failure of pyrantel has been reported from the Kimberley region of northwest Australia.[54]

Where appropriate, treat iron deficiency anaemia.

FOLLOW UP

Repeat faecal examinations 2–4 weeks post-therapy. If only a few eggs are observed in faecal concentrations, there is no need to repeat the therapy.

DRUG AVAILABILITY IN AUSTRALIA

Albendazole   *Eskazole:* 400 mg tabs
                  Zentel: 200 mg tabs
Mebendazole   *Banworm:* 100 mg tabs
                  Sqworm: 100 mg tabs
                  Vermox: 100 mg tabs; 100 mg/5 mL suspension
Pyrantel embonate   *Anthel:* 125 mg, 250 mg tabs
                        Combantrin: 125 mg, 250 mg tabs
                        Early Bird: 100 mg chocolate squares

Hymenolepis nana

Cestode: dwarf tapeworm

LIFE CYCLE AND EPIDEMIOLOGY

Hymenolepis nana is a unique cestode because the life cycle can be maintained between humans without an intermediate host. Spread is by faecal–oral transmission. The adult worm develops within the small intestine and begins egg production within 1 month. Eggs are immediately infective and can develop into larvae and mature within the intestinal wall (autoinfection), leading to amplification of the worm burden. The life span of an adult worm is 4–6 weeks, but internal autoinfection allows the infection to persist for years.

There is a worldwide distribution of infection and the prevalence is highest among children in areas where sanitation is poor.

CLINICAL NOTES

Patients may be asymptomatic or, in heavier infections, complain of anorexia, abdominal cramps and diarrhoea. Infections have usually cleared by adolescence and are uncommon in healthy adults.

DIAGNOSIS

* Demonstration of eggs in faecal specimens. Egg output may be intermittent or in low numbers, so examination of multiple specimens is essential. Adult worms and proglottids are rarely seen (see Plates 38, 39).
* Low-grade peripheral eosinophilia is common.

TREATMENT

Praziquantel   25 mg/kg single dose po (repeat after 1 week if heavy infestation)

or   **Niclosamide**
Children   11–34 kg: 1 g, chewed, then 0.5 g/day for 6 days
> 35 kg: 1.5 g, chewed, then 1 g/day for 6 days
Adults 2 g single dose, chewed, then 1 g/day for 6 days

FOLLOW UP

Repeat faecal examination for eggs at 1 and 3 months after therapy.

DRUG AVAILABILITY IN AUSTRALIA

Niclosamide *Yomesan:* not currently available in Australia
Praziquantel *Biltricide:* 600 mg tabs

Isospora belli

Intestinal coccidian protozoan

Isospora belli is acquired by ingestion of contaminated food or water. The parasites develop and multiply in the epithelial cells of the small intestine. Immature oocysts are excreted in the faeces and undergo further maturation before becoming infectious. Oocysts are highly resistant to adverse environmental conditions. Humans are the only known hosts.

The infection is endemic in certain areas in the tropics, and has been reported in central Australia. It is a rare cause of traveller's diarrhoea and an important, but uncommon, cause of diarrhoea in immunocompromised individuals.

CLINICAL NOTES

Infection usually causes mild, transient gastrointestinal symptoms in the immunocompetent host. These may include non-bloody diarrhoea with crampy abdominal pain, which can last for weeks and result in malabsorption and weight loss, especially in children. In immunosuppressed patients the watery diarrhoea is often profuse and protracted and associated with abdominal discomfort, malabsorption and low-grade fever. In AIDS patients it often leads to weakness, dehydration and weight loss.

DIAGNOSIS

Demonstration of the large, typical-shaped oocysts in faecal specimens. Multiple faecal samples should be examined using wet mounts or modified acid-fast staining, as the oocysts may be passed in small numbers and intermittently (see Plate 11). If stool examinations are negative, examine duodenal specimens from a biopsy or string test (Entero-Test).

> Specifically request *Isospora*, as diagnosis may be missed if only an egg or cyst examination is requested.

TREATMENT

Trimethoprim-sulfamethoxazole 160 mg TMP + 800 mg SMX (i.e. 1 DS tablet) four times daily po for 10 days, then twice daily for 3 weeks.

Long-term maintenance therapy may be required
in AIDS patients.

FOLLOW UP

Repeat faecal examinations 2–4 weeks after therapy to confirm
parasite clearance.

DRUG AVAILABILITY IN AUSTRALIA

Trimethoprim-sulfamethoxazole
 Bactrim or *Septrin* or *Resprim:* 80 mg, 400 mg tabs
 Bactrim DS or *Septrin Forte* or *Resprim Forte:* 160 mg, 800 mg tabs

Leishmania spp.

Obligate intracellular protozoa

LIFE CYCLE AND EPIDEMIOLOGY

Several species of *Leishmania* that cause different clinical manifestations are found in different geographical areas. Infection is transmitted by female sand-fly bites (*Phlebotomus* and *Lutzomia* spp.). Once within mammalian skin, promastigotes are rapidly taken up by macrophages and transform into intracellular amastigotes. Human leishmaniasis is a zoonosis (transmitted from domestic animals, rodents and dogs), except in India where humans are the only mammalian hosts. Inadequate sanitation and unsatisfactory housing facilitate transmission.

Leishmania spp. are opportunistic pathogens in HIV-infected patients. Visceral leishmaniasis (kala-azar) is caused primarily by the *L. donovani* complex (*L. donovani*, *L. infantum* and *L. chagasi*), and to a lesser extent by *L. tropica*, in the Old World, and by *L. amazonensis* in the New World. Several species may cause cutaneous leishmaniasis, depending on geographical location, including *L. tropica*, *L. major*, *L. braziliensis* and *L. mexicana*.

Visceral and cutaneous leishmaniasis are prevalent in China, India, the Middle East, Africa, southern Europe, and Central and South America.

CLINICAL NOTES

Leishmaniasis is rare in returned travellers. The incubation period is usually from 3 to 8 months (but may be 10 days to 14 years).[55] Many infections are asymptomatic or self-healing.

There are four main clinical syndromes depending on the species of leishmania, the geographical location and the host's immune response.

Visceral leishmaniasis (kala-azar) often presents with intermittent fever, hepatosplenomegaly, lymphadenopathy, anaemia, diarrhoea and progressive weight loss. In some cases, however, there is isolated splenomegaly with minimal symptoms. In the later stages of disease there is massive organomegaly, emaciation and discoloured (grey) skin. Bacterial superinfection is common. Atypical presentations occur in HIV-infected patients.

Post-kala-azar dermal leishmaniasis may follow treatment of visceral disease in persons in Africa and India. Skin lesions vary from depigmented or hyperpigmented macules to nodules lasting months (Africa) to years (India). This condition can mimic leprosy.

Cutaneous leishmaniasis ('oriental sore') is characterised by single or multiple lesions (papules, nodules and ulcers) that may last for many months. Scars are atrophic and depigmented.

Mucosal leishmaniasis is found in Central and South America. This form of leishmaniasis results in nasopharyngeal lesions that can be severe. Mutilating mucosal infection is typical of *L. braziliensis*. ENT examination may be required to detect early lesions.

DIAGNOSIS

* Microscopic examination of Giemsa-stained smears of tissue scrapings or aspirates, or biopsy material, for the presence of amastigotes.

  Visceral leishmaniasis Microscopic examination of aspirates of bone marrow and/or spleen and/or biopsies of liver or lymph node are carried out to demonstrate LD bodies (amastigote forms). Splenic aspirate has a 96–98% positivity rate, but should be performed by experienced personnel. Non-specific findings include normocytic, normochromic anaemia, leucopenia, thrombocytopenia and hypergammaglobulinaemia.

  Cutaneous leishmaniasis Diagnosis relies on identification of amastigotes in stained smears of scrapings, biopsies or aspirates of the base or the border of skin lesions (see Plate 5).

* Culture of buffy coat, aspirates, scrapings or biopsy material may be performed in special cases at the Walter and Eliza Hall Institute, Melbourne, or NNN medium is available for culture from CIDM, Westmead Hospital, Sydney. The different species are morphologically indistinguishable, but can be differentiated on the basis of their isoenzymes, antigens and nucleic acids.

* **Serology** Anti-leishmanial antibodies may be detected by IHA using *L. donovani* promastigote antigen (Sudan strain). In visceral disease, antibody titres may be seen in as little as 2 weeks post-infection. Circulating antibodies may be present in cutaneous leishmaniasis if the lymphatics and regional lymph nodes are involved. Cross-reactions occur with sera from patients with other parasitic infections, especially Chagas' disease, malaria, leprosy and schistosomiasis. An IFA can be performed at CIDM, Westmead Hospital, Sydney. Speciation is not possible using either IHA or IFA.

TREATMENT

The treatment of visceral and mucocutaneous leishmaniasis is complex and in the latter case depends on the likely species.[32,56]

General guidelines are given, but it is recommended that expert advice is sought and the treatment tailored to the individual case.

Visceral and mucocutaneous leishmaniasis:

> **Stibogluconate sodium** or **meglumine antimoniate**   20 mg of antimony/kg per day iv or im in a single dose or two divided doses for 28 days (up to 60 days if relapse occurs). Side effects are common. An ECG should be performed at the beginning of therapy and then weekly while on therapy. FBC, U&E and LFT should be monitored weekly.

If treatment with antimony compounds cannot be tolerated or has failed, try:

> **Amphotericin B**   0.5 mg/kg given daily by slow infusion for 1–3 months (total dose 0.65–1.5 g)

or **Liposomal amphotericin B** appears effective with fewer side effects[57]

> Immunocompetent patient: 1–1.5 mg/kg per day iv for 21 days
> Immunocompromised patient: 3 mg/kg per day iv for 10 days

or **Pentamidine isethionate**   2–4 mg/kg per day for at least 15 days. FBC, U&E and LFT should be monitored weekly.

Antimonials combined with allopurinol, pentamidine and amphotericin have been used successfully in refractory cases.

Antimony resistance has been reported from India. Amphotericin B is the drug of choice in resistant cases.[58]

Cutaneous leishmaniasis:

Treat only if lesions are large or disfiguring. First-line therapy is with **antimony compounds** for 20 days. Intralesional injection with antimony compounds has also been tried. Alternatively, in certain cases **itraconazole** may be used orally, in combination with antimony compounds, or alone although healing may be incomplete.[59] Oral **ketoconazole** is also effective for some species.[60] **Liposomal amphotericin B** has also been used. **Combination therapy** with local heat may be tried in diffuse cutaneous leishmaniasis.[61]

FOLLOW UP

Monitor the clinical and parasitological response to therapy. Serology may remain positive after chemotherapy. Relapses usually occur within 6 months and are more common in patients with concurrent HIV infection. Repeat bone marrow or splenic aspirates at 3 and 12 months after treatment are recommended for the early detection of relapses.

DRUG AVAILABILITY IN AUSTRALIA

Amphotericin B *Fungizone* intravenous: 50 mg vials

Itraconazole *Sporonox:* 100 mg caps

Ketoconazole *Nizoral:* 200 mg tabs

Liposomal amphotericin B *AmBisome:* 50 mg vials

Meglumine antimoniate [SAS approval] *Glucantim* (Contact Aventis for direct importation.)

Pentamidine *Pentamidine isethionate for injection* BP: 300 mg vials

Stibogluconate sodium [SAS approval]
  Pentostam: injection with 100 mg/mL of antimony (Contact Glaxo-Wellcome for direct importation.)

Loa loa

Filarial nematode: African eyeworm

LIFE CYCLE AND EPIDEMIOLOGY

Loa loa is transmitted by the bite of the deer fly or mango fly (*Chrysops* spp.). Adult worms live in the subcutaneous tissues. Sheathed microfilariae are found in blood and have a diurnal periodicity with the peak at midday.

The disease is seen in West and Central Africa (rainforest areas). It is occasionally seen in Australia in travellers returning from endemic areas.

CLINICAL NOTES

Symptoms are due to the migration of adult worms through the subcutaneous tissue or the eye. Patients may present with transient, migratory, subcutaneous swellings (calabar swellings), conjunctivitis, fever and/or eosinophilia. Swellings may be accompanied by pain, pruritis or urticaria and last for 1–3 days. Complications include cardiomyopathy, encephalopathy, nephropathy and pleural effusion. Asymptomatic infections occur, particularly in residents (i.e. semi-immune) in endemic areas.

DIAGNOSIS

- Loiasis is often a clinical diagnosis, as microfilariae may not appear in peripheral blood for years.
- Multiple peripheral blood examinations should be taken during the day (diurnal periodicity) to demonstrate microfilariae (wet preparation, microhaematocrit preparation, T+T smear including buffy coat, Knott concentration and membrane filtration are all useful techniques).
- Identification of the worm if removal from the eye or swelling is possible.
- **Serology** An EIA using heterologous antigens from the adult worm of the dog filarial species *Dirofilaria immitis* detects circulating antibodies. A highly positive result (i.e. OD > 1.00) suggests exposure, but low positive or borderline results are difficult to interpret. The false positivity rate is high (up to 30%) and cross-reactions with sera from patients with other nematode infections, especially strongyloidiasis, are common. Most people from an area of endemicity will have a positive serological result

from previous infection. This assay does not distinguish between filarial species.
• Peripheral eosinophilia is common.

TREATMENT

Surgical removal of the worm from the eye where possible.

Diethylcarbamazine
Day 1: 50 mg po, after food
Day 2: 50 mg three times daily
Day 3: 100 mg three times daily
Days 4–21: 9 mg/kg per day in 3 doses

or **Ivermectin** 200 µg/kg stat, repeat every 6–12 months.

Encephalitis, which is often fatal, may be precipitated by treatment if the microfilarial load is high, so **corticosteroids** should be administered with antifilarial drugs, and diethylcarbamazine (DEC) should be introduced gradually in these patients.

FOLLOW UP
Repeat blood smears for microfilariae 2–4 weeks after therapy.

DRUG AVAILABILITY IN AUSTRALIA

Diethylcarbamazine *Hetrazan:* 50 mg tabs
Ivermectin *Stromectol:* 6 mg tabs

Maggots (larval forms of flies or fleas)

Chrysomyia bezziana (Old World screw worm fly)
Cochliomyia hominivorax (New World screw worm fly)
Cordylobia anthropophaga (Tumbu fly)
Dermatobium hominis (botfly/tropical warble fly)
Tunga penetrans (jigger flea)
Oestrus ovis (sheep warble fly)

LIFE CYCLE AND EPIDEMIOLOGY

Deposition of either eggs or larvae is the probable mode of human infestation. The infection is occasionally encountered in Australian travellers[62] and in tropical areas of Australia.[63] Human infestation is often due to Tumbu fly (Africa) or botfly (Central and South America) and affected individuals usually give a history of travel to Africa, or South or Central America. Cases of acute conjunctival irritation from deposition of larvae of sheep warble fly are not infrequent in sheep rearing areas of Australia.

It is important to recognise and control the disease, as it could be a threat to agriculture and public health in Australia.

CLINICAL NOTES

Myiasis is the infestation of live human and vertebrate animals with dipterous (flies, mosquitos and relatives) larvae that feed on host tissue. Maggots can infest any accessible organ or tissue.

Cutaneous myiasis presents with an itchy swelling (sun spot, sore, pimple or boil) over the site of the bite. This may later bleed, but is seldom painful. Patients may complain of feeling 'something in the sore'. Sometimes a large subdermal itchy cyst (jiggers) may be seen, usually on the feet. The larvae of botflies may advance in the skin and mimic CLM.

Intestinal myiasis develops when eggs or larvae are accidentally deposited on food, and after ingestion these may irritate the intestinal mucosa.

Ophthalmomyiasis may present as acute irritation of the conjunctiva.

DIAGNOSIS

Confirmed by identifying the larvae after removal (see Plate 58).

> Larvae should be submitted to the local State Department of Agriculture or medical entomology facility for identification and documentation.

TREATMENT

Smear the wound with **petroleum jelly** to suffocate the maggots. Then remove them with forceps or a sterile needle.

Sometimes **surgical removal** may be necessary, taking care not to transect the larvae, which may lead to a severe inflammatory response. **Antibiotics** may be required if there is secondary bacterial infection.

Remove larvae from the conjunctivae by **irrigation** or under direct vision.

PREVENTION

Tumbu flies lay eggs on washed clothes. Travellers to endemic areas should be instructed to hang drip-dry clothes indoors with windows closed. All clothing and towels should be ironed on both sides.

FOLLOW UP

Watch for secondary bacterial infection.

Mansonella ozzardi

LIFE CYCLE AND EPIDEMIOLOGY

Mansonella ozzardi is transmitted by the bite of blackflies (*Simulium* spp.) and midges (*Culicoides* spp.) in Latin America and the West Indies. Humans are the only known reservoir hosts. Adult worms live in the subcutaneous and connective tissues and microfilariae are found in the blood and skin. The microfilariae are non-periodic and unsheathed.

CLINICAL NOTES

The infection is usually asymptomatic and some investigators question the pathogenicity of the organism. However, infection has been associated with fever, headache, severe joint pain (especially knees and ankles), lymphadenopathy, pruritis, urticaria and angioedema.

DIAGNOSIS

- Peripheral blood examination is required to demonstrate un-sheathed microfilariae (use wet preparation, microhaematocrit preparation, T+T smear including buffy coat, Knott concentration and membrane filtration). The thick blood film should be scanned at low magnification (×100–150), otherwise microfilariae can readily be missed.
- Also examine skin snips for microfilariae (see *Onchocerca volvulus*).
- **Serology** An EIA using heterologous antigens from the adult worm of the dog filarial species *Dirofilaria immitis* is available to detect circulating anti-filarial antibodies. A highly positive result (i.e. OD > 1.00) suggests exposure to filaria, but low positive or borderline results are difficult to interpret. The false positivity rate is high (up to 30%) and cross-reactions with sera from patients with other nematode infections, especially strongyloidiasis, are common. The test does not differentiate past infections from current, or between filarial species.
- Peripheral eosinophilia may occur.

TREATMENT

Asymptomatic individuals in endemic areas need not be treated.

Symptomatic cases should be treated with:

Ivermectin 150 µg/kg stat po.

Diethylcarbamazine is not effective.

FOLLOW UP

Repeat blood smears for microfilariae 2–4 weeks after therapy.

DRUG AVAILABILITY IN AUSTRALIA

Ivermectin *Stromectol:* 6 mg tabs

Mansonella perstans
(previously known as *Dipetalonema perstans*)

LIFE CYCLE AND EPIDEMIOLOGY

Mansonella perstans is transmitted by midges (*Culicoides* spp.) in central Africa (east to west coast), the West Indies and Central and South America. Humans and some other primates are the reservoir hosts. Adult worms are found in the peritoneal and pleural cavities and microfilariae are found in the blood. The microfilariae are non-periodic and unsheathed.

CLINICAL NOTES

The adult worms produce little or no host immune response and so infection is usually asymptomatic, although eosinophilia is common. Microfilaraemia has been associated with pruritis, urticaria, fever, calabar-like swellings, arthralgia, abdominal pain and conjunctival nodules.

DIAGNOSIS

- Peripheral blood examination is required to demonstrate unsheathed microfilariae (wet preparations, microhaematocrit preparation, T+T smears including buffy coat, Knott concentration and membrane filtration are all useful techniques). The thick blood film should be scanned at low magnification (×100–150), otherwise microfilariae can easily be missed.
- **Serology** An EIA using heterologous antigens from the adult worm of the dog filarial species *Dirofilaria immitis* is available for the detection of circulating antibodies. A highly positive result (i.e. OD > 1.00) suggests exposure, but low positive or borderline results are difficult to interpret. The false positivity rate is high (up

to 30%) and cross-reactions with sera from patients with other nematode infections, especially strongyloidiasis, are common. The EIA does not differentiate past infections from current, or between filarial species.

* Peripheral eosinophilia is common

TREATMENT

Mebendazole 100 mg twice daily po for 30 days.

Ivermectin and diethylcarbamazine are not effective.

FOLLOW UP

Repeat blood smears for microfilariae 2–4 weeks after therapy.

DRUG AVAILABILITY IN AUSTRALIA

Mebendazole   *Banworm:* 100 mg tabs
Sqworm: 100 mg tabs
Vermox: 100 mg tabs; 100 mg/5 mL suspension

Mansonella streptocerca
(previously known as *Dipetalonema streptocerca*)

LIFE CYCLE AND EPIDEMIOLOGY

Mansonella streptocerca is transmitted by biting midges (*Culicoides* spp.) in the Congo basin area of West Africa. Humans and monkeys are the reservoir hosts. The adult worms live in the dermal tissues of the upper thorax and shoulders and microfilariae are found in the skin. The microfilariae are unsheathed.

CLINICAL NOTES

The infection is usually asymptomatic, but may cause pruritic dermatitis, hypopigmented macules and papules, with associated lymphadenopathy. Some reports suggest that the skin manifestations are most marked over the thorax and shoulders. Inguinal lymphadenopathy is common.

DIAGNOSIS

* Microscopic detection of unsheathed microfilariae in skin snips. Multiple skin snips (especially from the shoulder region) should be taken. These microfilariae need to be differentiated from the unsheathed microfilariae of *Onchocerca volvulus*.

- **Serology** As for the other filaria, an EIA using heterologous antigens from the adult worm of the dog filarial species *Dirofilaria immitis* is available for the detection of circulating antibodies. A highly positive result (i.e. OD > 1.00) suggests exposure, but low positive or borderline results are difficult to interpret. The false positivity rate is high (up to 30%) and cross-reactions with sera from patients with other nematode infections, especially strongyloidiasis, are common. The EIA does not differentiate past infections from current, or between filarial species.
- Peripheral eosinophilia may occur.

TREATMENT

Diethylcarbamazine
Day 1: 50 mg po, after food
Day 2: 50 mg three times daily
Day 3: 100 mg three times daily
Days 4–21: 6 mg/kg per day in 3 doses

The treatment may be associated with intense pruritis.

> **The efficacy of ivermectin is unproven.**

FOLLOW UP

Repeat skin snip examinations if symptoms persist or recur.

DRUG AVAILABILITY IN AUSTRALIA

Diethylcarbamazine *Hetrazan:* 50 mg tabs

Microsporidia

Protozoa: several genera cause human diseases.

Enterocytozoon: *E. bieneusi*
Encephalitozoon: *E. cuniculi*, *E. hellem*, *E. (Septata) intestinalis*
Nosema: *N. connori*, *N. ocularum*
Pleistophora spp.
Vittaforma: *V. corneae* (previously *N. corneum*)
Trachipleistophora: *T. hominis*
Microsporidium: *M. ceylonensis*, *M. africanum*

LIFE CYCLE AND EPIDEMIOLOGY

More than 100 genera and 1000 species of intracellular protozoan parasites belonging to the phylum Microsporidia have been described. They infect every major animal group, and at least seven species are well characterised as human pathogens.

Microsporidia are characterised by the production of resistant spores measuring 1–4 μm, depending on the species. They possess a unique organelle, the polar tubule or polar filament, which is coiled inside the spore. The resistant spore is the infective form, which hatches by extruding its polar tubule and infecting the host cell. Inside the cell, the sporoplasm undergoes multiplication and maturation to form mature spores. When the spores completely fill the host cell cytoplasm, the cell membrane is disrupted and releases the spores to the surroundings. These free, mature spores can infect new cells thus continuing the cycle, or persist for long periods in the environment. Person-to-person and animal-to-human transmission are postulated.

Sero-epidemiology studies show worldwide distribution, but probably have limited value due to a high rate of cross-reactivity. There is a much higher incidence of disease in immunocompromised patients (especially AIDS patients).

CLINICAL NOTES

Microsporidiosis is an important opportunistic infection occurring predominantly in severely immunocompromised patients with AIDS. There have been isolated case reports since 1959 of CNS, corneal, muscle and gastrointestinal disease in both immunocompromised patients who are not infected with HIV and immunocompetent patients.[64]

The clinical manifestations vary with the species:

Enterocytozoon bieneusi Chronic diarrhoea, anorexia and weight loss are common. Cholangitis and respiratory tract involvement also occur.

Encephalitozoon hellem, E. cuniculi Keratoconjunctivitis that is usually bilateral. Systemic disease, including bronchiolitis, sinusitis, nephritis, cystitis, hepatitis and peritonitis, also occurs.

E. intestinalis (Septata) may cause diarrhoea and wasting as well as biliary disease. Occassionally it disseminates to the eye, kidney, lungs and nasal sinuses.

Pleistophora spp. Rare, but muscle involvement has been reported.

Vittaforma and *Nosema* spp. Rare, but corneal involvement has been reported.

Trachipleistophora hominis Myositis was recently reported in an Australian patient.[65]

Microsporidium ceylonensis, M. africanum Rare, but infection of the cornea has been reported.

DIAGNOSIS

- Light microscopic examination of stained smears of clinical specimens is the easiest method of diagnosis. A variety of stains can be used, including Ryan's stain.[66] The type of clinical specimens collected will depend on the symptoms, but may include BAL, conjunctival smears, urine (some species), and NPA. The spores of *Enterocytozoon bieneusi* measure 0.8–1.4 µm and those of *Encephalitozoon* spp., *Vittaforma corneae* and *Nosema* spp. measure 1.5–4 µm (see Plates 8–10).
- Transmission electron microscopy (TEM) is still the method of choice for distinguishing between the microsporidia. However, TEM is usually only used in reference laboratories.
- PCR diagnosis is becoming increasingly available, but at present it remains a research tool.

TREATMENT

Albendazole 400 mg twice daily po for 28 days appears effective for *Encephalitozoon* and *Trachipleistophora* infections, including disseminated disease.[65,67,68] May be effective in other microsporidia.

Octreotide is a useful palliative agent for refractory diarrhoea. Give 50 mg sc, increasing the dose slowly in 100 mg increments until a response is obtained (max. 500 mg/day).

Fumagillin B drops and **propamidine isethionate** (1%) are effective for *Encephalitozoon* corneal infections. Prolonged therapy is required.

FOLLOW UP

Monitor the clinical course and parasite load, depending on the symptoms.

DRUG AVAILABILITY IN AUSTRALIA

Albendazole *Eskazole:* 400 mg tabs
                 Zentel: 200 mg tabs
Fumagillin B not currently available in Australia
Octreotide *Sandostatin:* 0.05, 0.1 and 0.5 mg/mL ampoules
Propamidine 0.1% *Brolene* eye drops

Naegleria fowleri

Protozoan: free-living amoeba in fresh water or moist soil

LIFE CYCLE AND EPIDEMIOLOGY

Naegleria fowleri is found in natural, fresh, warm water collections such as artesian hot springs, especially where the water is in direct contact with soil. The trophozoites may invade the CNS (via the olfactory nerve) of children and young adults who swim or dive in contaminated water. Unlike *Acanthamoeba* spp., there is no cyst form of *N. fowleri* in human infections. The infection is rare, but there is a worldwide distribution.

CLINICAL NOTES

Primary amoebic meningoencephalitis has an incubation period of 3–7 days. Early manifestations include fever, severe headache, neck stiffness, sore throat and rhinitis. The illness is often mistaken for bacterial meningitis, but progresses over subsequent days in spite of antibiotic treatment. The patient has a rising fever, worsening headache, and develops focal neurological deficits, coma and dies within approximately 10 days. A CT scan may show basal arachnoiditis.

DIAGNOSIS

- The CSF may be purulent or haemorrhagic and the pressure is often elevated. There is marked leucocytosis, decreased glucose, increased protein, and no bacteria seen on Gram stain.
- Microscopic examination of a wet mount of CSF for amoeboid trophozoites, which have a spherical nucleus and a large karyosome (easily confused with leucocytes). A Giemsa-stained smear may also show trophozoites with typical morphology.
- Organisms can be cultured on 1.5% non-nutrient agar overlaid with *E. coli*.
- Trophozoites, but not cysts, may also be found in tissue specimens (compare with *Acanthamoeba* spp.).

Do not refrigerate specimens prior to examination.

TREATMENT

Early diagnosis and treatment is critical, as recovery is rare.[17,69]

Amphotericin B 1 mg/kg per day iv, and intraventricular (via a reservoir), 0.1–1 mg on alternate days.

The duration of therapy is uncertain.

Combination therapy with **miconazole** and **rifampicin** has been tried with some success.

Dexamethasone and **antiepileptics** are used as necessary.

FOLLOW UP

Monitor the clinical response and the number of organisms in the CSF using direct wet mounts and cultures.

DRUG AVAILABILITY IN AUSTRALIA

Amphotericin B *Fungizone* intravenous: 50 mg vials

Onchocerca volvulus

Filarial nematode

LIFE CYCLE AND EPIDEMIOLOGY

Infection is transmitted by the bite of the blackfly (*Simulium* spp.). Adult worms develop in the skin and subcutaneous nodules over several months. They then begin releasing microfilariae, which are found in the skin 7–34 months following infection.

Most cases occur in equatorial Africa (particularly West Africa); a few cases occur in Guatemala and Mexico and the northern part of South America. There is a higher incidence in people living along rivers and streams because the vector deposits eggs into free-flowing water, particularly in rapids. The fly usually bites during the day. *Onchocerca volvulus* infection is unusual in travellers unless there is heavy and/or prolonged exposure.

CLINICAL NOTES

The main features of **onchocerciasis** are dermatitis, eye lesions and subcutaneous nodules, although many infected individuals are asymptomatic. Early features include intense itch and an erythematous, papular rash, fever and musculoskeletal pains. Later, subcutaneous nodules (painless and measuring a few millimetres or centimetres), leathery, dyspigmented skin (leopard skin), lymphadenopathy, punctate keratitis, chorioretinitis, and optic atrophy may develop (hence the disease is also called 'river blindness'). Skin and eye lesions are variable depending on the geographic area. A condition called 'Sowdah' exists in certain areas and is characterised by intense pruritis, darkened scaly skin and lymphadenopathy. The pruritic skin rash needs to be distinguished from scabies.

DIAGNOSIS

- Demonstration of unsheathed microfilariae in multiple skin snips from the scapulae and deltoids (if acquired in Central or South America) or iliac crests, buttocks and thighs (if acquired in Africa) as well as one snip from the skin covering any nodules. If microfilariae cannot be demonstrated, test for a Mazzoti reaction (single oral dose of 50 mg DEC leads to pruritis and exacerbation of rash within 0.5–24 hours). Differentiate from the smaller microfilariae of *Mansonella streptocerca*, which are also found in the skin.

- Histopathological examination of an excised nodule may reveal the adult worm.
- Slit-lamp examination of the eye may detect microfilariae in the anterior chamber or cornea.
- Ultrasonography may detect deep non-palpable onchocercal nodules.[70]
- **Serology** As for the other filaria, an EIA is available. A highly positive result (i.e. OD > 1.00) suggests exposure, but low positive or borderline results are difficult to interpret. The false positivity rate is high (up to 30%) and cross-reactions with sera from patients with other nematode infections are common. Most people from an area of endemicity will have a positive serological result. The EIA does not distinguish between filarial species.
- Eosinophilia is common.

TREATMENT

Ivermectin 150 µg/kg stat po, repeat every 6–12 months. Kills microfilariae, but has little effect on adult worms. Repeated treatment every 3–6 months for 2–3 years or longer may eventually eradicate the infection.[17]

Surgical removal of nodules is effective in reducing the adult worm burden.

> Monitor for treatment reactions. These are milder with ivermectin than with DEC and include fever, pruritis, and urticaria. Aspirin may be useful for reducing these effects.
>
> Oral corticosteroids (1 mg/kg per day) may be given for several days before starting ivermectin if eye infection is present.
>
> Treatment with DEC is not recommended because of the frequency of severe reactions.

FOLLOW UP

Skin snips should be repeated 3 monthly after treatment to ensure clearance of microfilariae. Re-treat every 6–12 months or earlier if symptoms return.

DRUG AVAILABILITY IN AUSTRALIA

Ivermectin *Stromectol:* 6 mg tabs

Opisthorchis (Clonorchis) spp.

Trematodes: liver flukes

LIFE CYCLE AND EPIDEMIOLOGY

Human infection is acquired by eating raw or inadequately cooked freshwater fish that contains the infective larval form (metacercariae). After ingestion, the larvae migrate through the ampulla of Vater into the biliary and pancreatic ducts and mature into adult flukes and begin egg production in about 4 weeks. Eggs are passed in the faeces and may contaminate fresh water. After ingestion by a snail inter-mediate host, the eggs release miracidia, which undergo further devel-opment in the snail. Free-swimming cercariae are then released and invade certain fish species (second intermediate host) and form metacercaria. The mammalian definitive host (cats, dogs, and various fish-eating mammals including humans) becomes infected by ingesting undercooked fish containing metacercariae. Humans, dogs, cats and other fish-eating mammals may also act as reservoir hosts. Frozen, pickled or dried fish is also implicated in transmission.

Opisthorchis sinensis is known as the Oriental or Chinese liver fluke and is most common in China, Hong Kong, Japan, Taiwan, Vietnam and Korea. *Opisthorchis felineus* (cat liver fluke) and *O. viverrini* (South East Asian liver fluke) are also acquired by eating inadequately cooked fish and produce an illness similar to that of *O. sinensis*. *Opisthorchis felineus* is endemic in South East Asia and eastern Europe, and *O. viverrini* in north-eastern Thailand, Cambodia and Laos.

CLINICAL NOTES

Most patients are asymptomatic early in the infection. Mild symptoms (associated with 100–1000 worms) include epigastric or RUQ abdominal discomfort, anorexia, nausea and diarrhoea lasting days to weeks. With a heavy worm burden, abdominal pain worsens and both the liver and gall-bladder enlarge. Cholecystitis, recurrent cholangitis, pancreatitis and obstructive jaundice may occur. There is a strong association with hepatic cirrhosis and cholangiocarcinoma. Passage of eggs may continue for decades after infection.

DIAGNOSIS

- Microscopic demonstration of eggs in faeces, bile or duodenal contents. Multiple specimens should be examined to detect light infections. Concentration techniques are required to detect a low egg burden. The eggs of *O. sinensis* are difficult to distinguish from those of other *Opisthorchis* species (see Plate 32).

- CT scan or ultrasound imaging may identify flukes within the bile ducts.

TREATMENT

Praziquantel 25 mg/kg three times daily po for 1–2 days.

FOLLOW UP

Faecal examinations for eggs at 1 and 3 months after therapy.

DRUG AVAILABILITY IN AUSTRALIA

Praziquantel *Biltricide:* 600 mg tabs

Paragonimus mexicanus
Paragonimus westermani

Trematodes: lung flukes

LIFE CYCLE AND EPIDEMIOLOGY

Paragonimus spp. inhabit the lungs of some mammals (especially cats, but also dogs, monkeys and primates). Eggs expectorated or passed in the faeces in the vicinity of lakes or streams infect freshwater snails, which act as the first intermediate host. Cercariae may enter the second intermediate host (i.e. crabs, shrimp or crayfish) and humans acquire infection by ingesting raw or pickled crayfish or freshwater crabs. The metacercariae excyst in the duodenum and migrate via the peritoneal cavity and the diaphragm to the lungs. Here they become encapsulated and develop into adults and begin egg production 2–3 months after infection. The eggs are excreted in the sputum, or alternatively they are swallowed and passed with the stool. Occasionally ectopic migration occurs to the brain, heart, abdomen or skin. Infections may persist for 20 years in humans.

Paragonimus westermani occurs in India, China, South East Asia (especially Philippines, Laos and Thailand) and Africa; *P. mexicanus* occurs in Central and South America.

CLINICAL NOTES

Infections in which there is a low worm burden are asymptomatic. In the acute phase (invasion and migration), diarrhoea, abdominal pain, fever, cough, urticaria, hepatosplenomegaly, pulmonary abnormalities, and eosinophilia may occur. A productive cough with brown sputum and intermittent haemoptysis, and increasing chest pain may occur as the pulmonary cysts (i.e. the fibrotic capsule around the adult worm) rupture. Night sweats are also common. Eventually the disease progresses to chronic bronchitis or bronchiectasis with profuse sputum production and dyspnoea. Pulmonary tuberculosis is an important differential diagnosis.

Rarely, extrapulmonary locations of the adult worms result in more severe disease, including cerebral involvement (resembling epilepsy, tumour and infarction). These manifestations are more likely to occur in a younger age group. *Paragonimus westermani* is a cause of eosinophilic meningitis.

DIAGNOSIS

* Microscopic demonstration of eggs in faecal or sputum specimens. These are not present until 2–3 months after infection. Concentration techniques may be necessary in patients with light infections. Tissue biopsy may allow diagnostic confirmation and species identification when an adult fluke is recovered.
* CXR and CT imaging of the lung may be diagnostic, showing nodular shadows, patchy infiltration and cavities.
* Serology is available at CDC, Atlanta.
* Peripheral eosinophilia is common (20–25% of WCC).

TREATMENT

Praziquantel 25 mg/kg three times daily po for 3 days. Use in conjunction with **corticosteroids** in CNS infections.

FOLLOW UP

Sputum examination for eggs 2–4 weeks after therapy; faecal examinations for eggs 1–2 months after therapy. Monitor CXR and eosinophil count.

DRUG AVAILABILITY IN AUSTRALIA

Praziquantel *Biltricide:* 600 mg tabs

Pediculus spp.

Insecta: lice

Pediculus capitis (head louse)

LIFE CYCLE AND EPIDEMIOLOGY

Pediculus capitis is an ectoparasite that needs to feed on blood several times daily and requires the warmth of close contact with the scalp to maintain its body temperature. Transmission occurs by close contact, usually head-to-head transfer. Fomites can also transmit infection. This occurs by wearing infested clothing, such as hats and scarves, or by using infested combs, brushes or towels. Eggs (nits) are cemented at the base of the hair shaft, and 5–8 eggs are produced every day. The egg hatches releasing a nymph that looks like, but is smaller than, an adult head louse. Nymphs hatch out in 7–8 days, becoming adults in another 7–10 days. Adult lice can live up to 30 days on a person's head.

There is a higher incidence in school-age children, especially girls (longer hair and closer contact) and in daycare centres and institution settings. There is a worldwide distribution.

CLINICAL NOTES

There are usually no noticeable signs or symptoms although mild pruritis may occur. In heavy infestation severe pruritis of the scalp may occur. Scratching may then lead to excoriations and secondary bacterial infection with crusting and tender lymphadenopathy. Nits are visible at the base of hair shafts, particularly in the temporal and occipital areas.

DIAGNOSIS

Finding a live nymph or adult louse on the scalp or in the hair. Finding eggs (nits) is also highly suggestive of active infestation.

TREATMENT

Permethrin 1% Apply to hair, allow to remain for 10 minutes, then rinse off and comb the hair. Follow the label instructions.

or **Pyrethrin** Apply to dry hair, allow to remain for 10 minutes, then rinse and comb the hair. Follow the label instructions.

or **Maldison** Apply to hair, allow to remain for 10 minutes, then rinse off and comb the hair. Follow the label instructions.

Resistance has been reported in Australia recently.[71] Repeat with different active chemical if initial treatment does not work.

> It is important to wash in hot water all clothing and bed linen that have been in contact with the infested person in the 2 days before treatment. All household contacts should be checked for lice and nits every 2–3 days and treated if lice and nits are found. For children under 2 years of age, it may be preferable to remove nits and lice by hand.

A head lice information sheet for the public is available on the internet.[71]

FOLLOW UP

Examine hair 1 week after treatment. Re-treat if necessary.

DRUG AVAILABILITY IN AUSTRALIA

Maldison 0.5% *Cleensheen*
             Lice Rid
Permethrin 1% *Nix Creme Rinse*
             Pyrifoam shampoo
             Quellada Creme Rinse
             Quellada Head Lice Treatment
Pyrethrins + piperonyl butoxide *Banlice Mousse*

Pediculus humanis (*corporis*) (body louse)

LIFE CYCLE AND EPIDEMIOLOGY

This infestation is associated with poor personal hygiene. Transmission is through close contact with an infected person or with contaminated clothing or bedding. Eggs cement to cloth fibres or sometimes to body hair. The life cycle is similar to *P. capitis* and there is similarly a worldwide distribution.

> *Pediculus humanis* also transmits certain Rickettsial infections in endemic areas.

CLINICAL NOTES

Pruritis, erythematous macules, papules and excoriations are mainly found on the trunk. Secondary bacterial infection may occur as a result of scratching. Chronic infection may lead to depigmented, thickened skin ('vagabond's disease').

Pediculus spp.

DIAGNOSIS

The louse is not seen on the skin except in severe infections. In these cases the louse can be demonstrated in skin scrapings. Usually the louse can be found in the seams of clothing.

TREATMENT

Pyrethrin Apply to body, allow to remain for 10 minutes, before washing. Follow label instructions.

or **Benzyl benzoate** Apply to body, allow to remain for 24 hours before washing with soap and water.

Treat secondary bacterial infection with appropriate **antibiotics**.

In many cases it is only necessary to treat clothing and bedding by washing in hot water and then ironing the seams with a hot iron.

FOLLOW UP

Examine and treat clothing and bedding for nits and lice. Repeat treatment after 7 days if required.

DRUG AVAILABILITY IN AUSTRALIA

Benzyl benzoate 25% oil in water emulsion *Ascabiol*
Pyrethrins + piperonyl butoxide in a foaming base *Lyban Foam*

Phthirus pubis

Insecta: pubic or 'crab' louse

Pubic lice can be classified as an STD as transmission is by direct skin-to-skin transfer. Adult lice deposit and cement eggs to the pubic hair shafts, on which the shells remain attached after hatching. The life cycle is similar to *Pediculus capitis*. There is a worldwide distribution.

CLINICAL NOTES

Pubic, axillary and truncal hair, beard and eyelashes may all be involved, but the scalp is not. Pruritis may be severe. Erythematous macules, papules with excoriations and secondary bacterial infection are not as marked as those seen with *P. capitis* and *P. humanis*. Small bluish macules may occur on trunk, upper arms and thighs ('maculae cerulae') at the site of louse bites.

DIAGNOSIS

Microscopic demonstration of nits and occasionally adult lice at the base of affected hairs. Adult lice have massive claws, which differentiates them from *P. capitis* and *P. humanis*.

TREATMENT

Permethrin 1% Apply to pubic hair and other hair-bearing areas, allow to remain for 10 minutes, then rinse off. Follow the label instructions.

or **Pyrethrins** Apply to pubic hair and other hair-bearing areas, allow to remain for 10 minutes, then rinse off. Follow the label instructions.

Neither treatment can be used on eyelashes. Use petroleum jelly instead.

Remove nits carefully from eyelashes with forceps.

Wash clothing, especially underwear, and bed clothing and bedding in hot soapy water.

Treat secondary bacterial infection with an appropriate antibiotic.

FOLLOW UP

Check hair for nits and lice and re-treat in 1 week if necessary. Treat sexual contacts.

DRUG AVAILABILITY IN AUSTRALIA

Permethrin 1% *Quellada Creme Rinse*

Pyrethrins + piperonyl butoxide in kerosene in a foaming base *Lyban Foam*

Plasmodium spp.

Blood protozoa: malarial parasites

LIFE CYCLE AND EPIDEMIOLOGY

There are four species of *Plasmodium* that cause human malaria: *P. falciparum*, *P. vivax*, *P. ovale* and *P. malariae*. All are transmitted by the bite of the night-biting female *Anopheles* mosquito. Parasites develop to the schizont stage in the liver in 7–10 days (exoerythrocytic stage) and then the schizonts rupture, releasing merozoites into the bloodstream. In *P. vivax* and *P. ovale*, some parasites may become dormant in the liver (hypnozoites) and emerge at a later stage (up to 5 years after leaving an endemic area) to cause a relapse of the disease. Merozoites rapidly invade erythrocytes and develop into mature blood schizonts. New merozoites are released into the blood as the schizonts rupture (erythrocytic stage). The cycle repeats itself every 36–72 hours, depending on the species of *Plasmodium*. Multiplication of the erythrocytic-stage parasites is responsible for the clinical manifestations of the disease. In the blood, some parasites differentiate into the sexual erythrocytic stage (gametocytes). After ingestion by an *Anopheles* mosquito, the gametocytes undergo a sporogonic cycle yielding sporozoites. Inoculation of the sporozoites into a new human host completes the malaria life cycle.

In *P. falciparum* infections, erythrocytes containing mature parasite forms are sequestered in small blood vessels of organs such as brain, lung and placenta, which is the reason that only immature 'ring' forms of *P. falciparum* are seen in the peripheral blood, and is a major contributor to the pathology of this disease.

There are an estimated 270 million cases annually worldwide. In developed countries malaria is mainly seen in returned travellers from endemic countries. In Australia, 'airport malaria' has been reported[72] and outbreaks of introduced malaria occur in the Torres Strait Islands.

Plasmodium falciparum

CLINICAL NOTES

Patients usually present with fever and headache, but may have a variety of other presenting symptoms including cough, myalgia, arthralgia, abdominal pain, nausea, vomiting, diarrhoea, photophobia and altered conscious state. The fever may occur every 48 hours or continuously with intermittent peaks, and episodes may consist of cold with shaking, and hot and sweating phases. Splenomegaly is common and tachycardia, tachypnoea, icterus, pallor, hepatomegaly and hypotension occur. The clinical presentation can vary substantially depending on the level of parasitaemia, and the immune status of the patient.

> Suspect malaria in any traveller with fever who has been in an endemic area in the past 6–12 months, even if chemoprophylaxis was used.

P. falciparum malaria may develop complications and progress rapidly to death. Specific complications include cerebral malaria, severe anaemia, pulmonary oedema, and renal failure. A particular form of the latter is known as 'black water fever' due to the black urine caused by massive haemolysis. CNS manifestations may be due to cerebral malaria and/or hypoglycaemia.

DIAGNOSIS

- Demonstration of intraerythrocytic ring stage parasites in T+T blood smears (see Plate 24).

> At least three T+T smears taken 8–12 hours apart are required to exclude the diagnosis of malaria.

- A rapid diagnostic antigen test (immunochromatographic) is now available for *P. falciparum* and is often performed in parallel with microscopy (e.g. Amrad-ICT Malaria P.f.). The ICT has a sensitivity of 96% and a specificity of 90%.[73]
- Malaria PCR is available in some laboratories for use in difficult cases with low parasitaemia, possible mixed infections and uncertain parasite speciation.
- **Serology** is not appropriate for use in the diagnosis of acute malaria and should be used as a screen only. However, in areas where malaria is not endemic, serology may be useful for retrospective diagnosis in patients thought to have had malaria and who received therapy, and for the exclusion of malaria in patients with chronic or recurrent febrile illness. In areas where malaria is endemic, serology is of limited use because most of the population will have antibodies. An IFA assay using *P. falciparum* infected erythrocytes is available at CIDM, Westmead Hospital, Sydney.

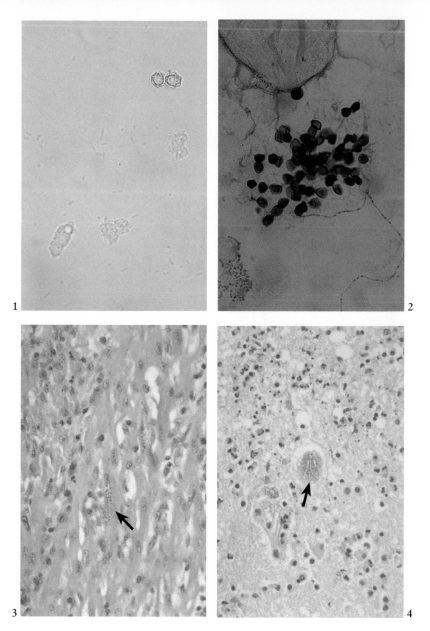

1 *Acanthamoeba* spp. cysts and trophozoites cultured from corneal scrapings. Direct microscopy of a non-nutrient agar plate (*Escherichia coli* seen in background). Cysts are typically double layered and stellate. Trophozoites have fine pseudopodia (called acanthopodia).

2 *Pneumocystis carinii* 'cysts' in induced sputum. Toludine blue stain. An immunoflorescent stain is also available.

3, 4 *Toxoplasma gondii* in an immunocompromised patient. Bradyzoites [3] in heart muscle, [4] in brain. H & E stain.

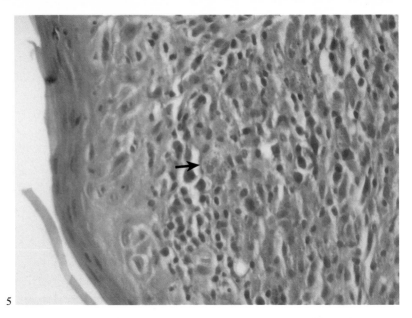

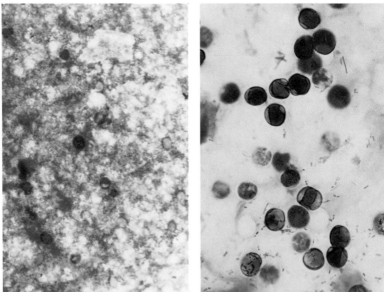

5 *Leishmania* spp. LD bodies (amastigote forms of the parasite) in skin biopsy in a patient with cutaneous leishmaniasis who had travelled to an endemic region. H & E stain.

6 *Cryptosporidium parvum* oocysts in faeces. Modified acid fast staining. These are usually about 4–5 μm in size.

7 *Cyclospora cayetanensis* oocysts in faeces. Modified acid fast staining. These are usually about 8–10 μm in size.

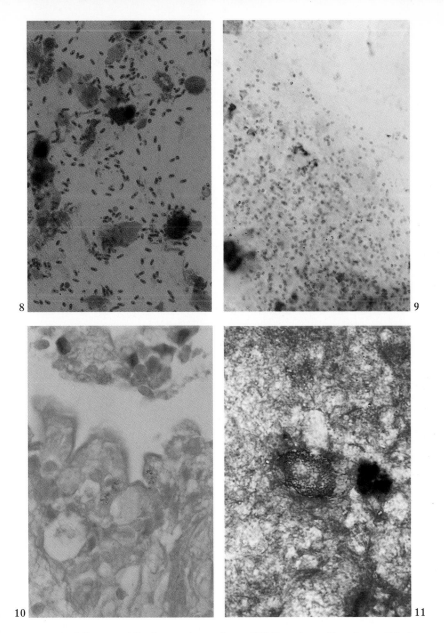

8, 9, 10 Microsporidia in specimen from AIDS patient. Ryan's modified trichrome stain. [8] *Encephalitozoon (Septata) intestinalis* in nasopharyngeal aspirate. Note the central band across the parasite. [9] *Enterocytozoon bieneusi* in urine. Note the large intracellular vacuole. [10] *Enterocytozoon bieneusi* in gall bladder tissue.

11 *Isospora belli* oocyst. Modified acid fast staining of faeces. Characteristically ovoid in shape and 20–33 × 10–19 µm in size.

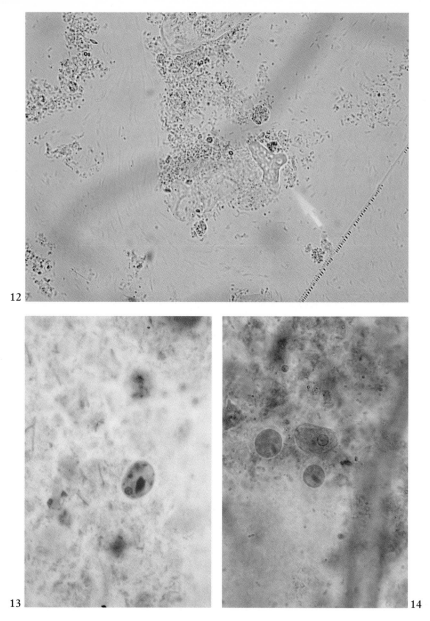

12, 13, 14 *Entamoeba histolytica* in faeces: [12] trophozoite, saline wet preparation; [13] cyst, trichrome stain; [14] trophozoite and cyst, iron-haematoxylin stain. This parasite can be confused with the non-pathogenic *Entamoeba coli* and should be differentiated from it by its nuclear and cytoplasmic features.

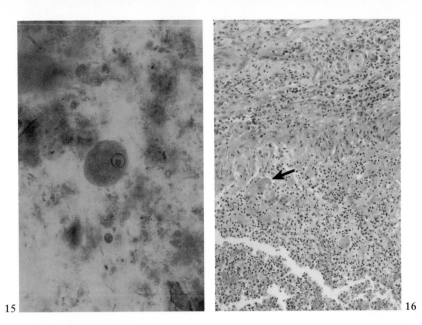

15

16

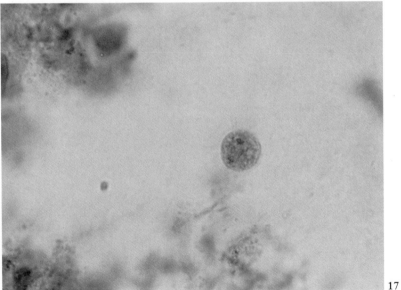

17

15 *Entamoeba coli* cyst in faeces. Iron-haematoxylin stain.

16 *Entamoeba histolytica* trophozoite in large intestine of a patient with amoebiasis. H & E stain.

17 *Dientamoeba fragilis* trophozoite in faeces. Iron-haematoxylin stain. Note the characteristic 'binucleate' nature of the nucleus, although a uninucleate form may also be seen. The morphology can be very varied. Cyst stage is not described for this parasite.

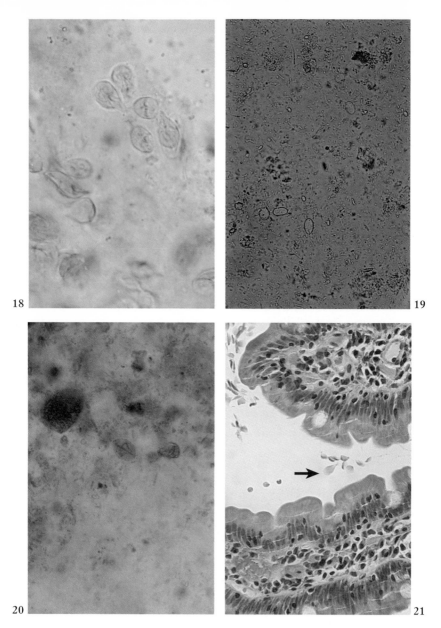

18, 19, 20 *Giardia duodenalis* in faeces: [18] trophozoites which have a typical 'face-like' appearance, iodine preparation; [19] cysts, saline wet preparation [20] cyst, iron-haematoxylin stain.

21 *Giardia duodenalis* trophozoites in lumen of small bowel. H & E stain.

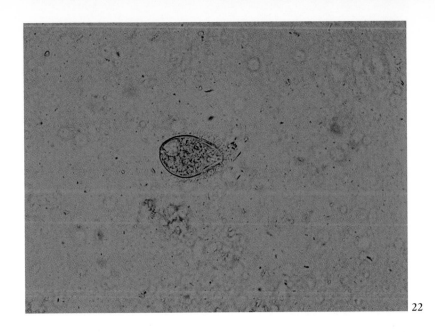

22

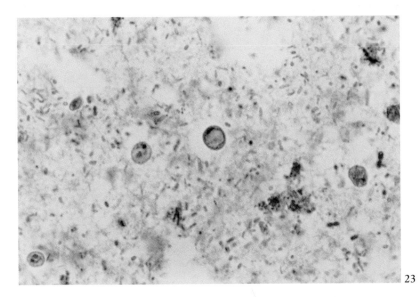

23

22 *Balantidium coli* trophozoite in faeces. Iodine preparation. This organism is recognised by its large size, prominent cytostome and ciliated surface.

23 *Blastocystis hominis* cysts in faeces. Iron-haematoxylin stain. The central mass with peripheral granules helps differentiate it from other protozoan cysts.

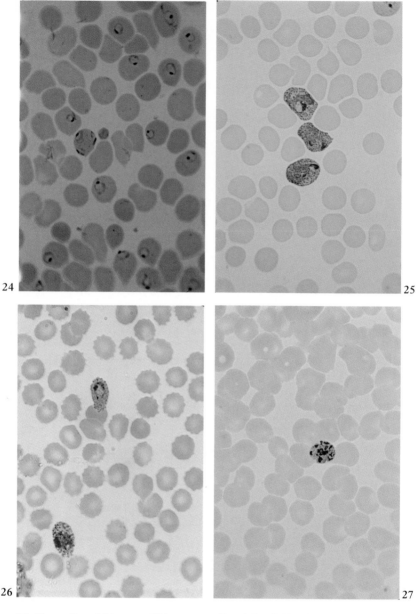

24 *Plasmodium falciparum.* Thin smear of peripheral blood showing multiple ring forms.

25 *Plasmodium vivax.* Thin smear of peripheral blood showing schizonts.

26 *Plasmodium ovale.* Thin smear of peripheral blood showing a ring form and a trophozoite. Note the oval shape of the affected red cells.

27 *Plasmodium malariae.* Thin smear of peripheral blood showing a schizont. Note the normal size of the affected red cell.

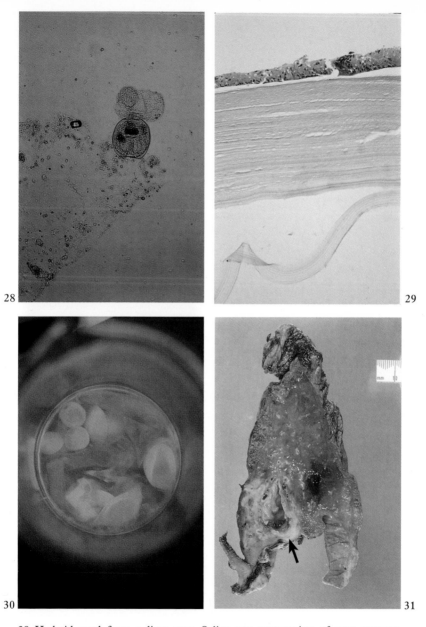

28 Hydatid sand from a liver cyst. Saline wet preparation of cyst contents showing a protoscolex (arrow) with an invaginated scolex and row of hooklets.

29 Hydatid cyst cross-section showing the outer laminated membrane. H & E stain.

30 Hydatid cyst surgically removed and displaying numerous daughter cysts of varying sizes.

31 Section of lung showing hydatid cyst in the lower lobe.

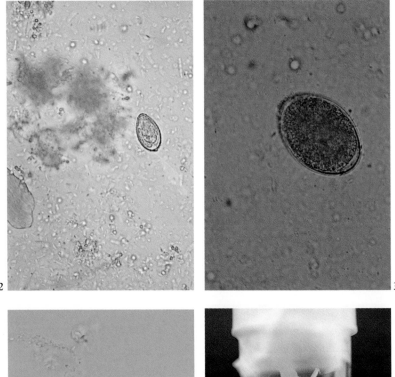

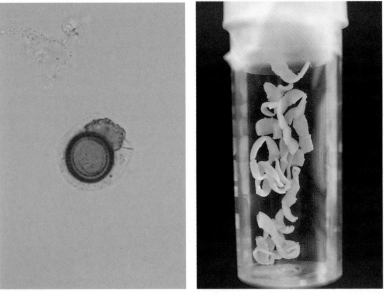

32 *Opisthorchis (Clonorchis) sinensis* eggs in faeces. Saline wet preparation. This is
diagnosed by its small size (≈ 30 μm) and the characteristic operculated egg
and small knobs at the end opposite the operculum.

33 *Diphyllobothrium latum* eggs in faeces. Saline wet preparation. The operculated
egg is characteristic and is differentiated from similar eggs by its size (58–
75 μm × 40–50 μm).

34, 35 *Taenia* spp. [34] Egg in faeces. Saline wet preparation. Note the striated
outer layer and three pairs of hooklets. The outer membranous capsule may not
always be present. [35] Part of adult worm passed in faeces after treatment.
Note the flat and segmented body. The number of uterine branches in a mature
proglottid (not shown here) differentiates the species.

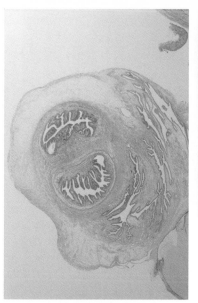

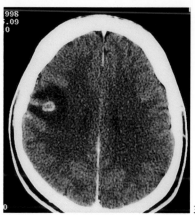

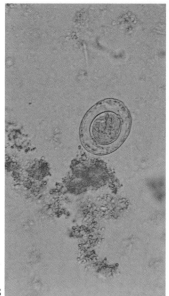

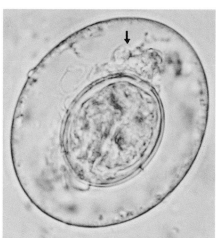

36 Biopsy of a skin nodule in a case of cutaneous cysticercosis, showing the larval (cystic) form of *Taenia solium*. H & E stain.

37 MRI of brain showing an active lesion in a case of neurocysticercosis.

38, 39 *Hymenolepis nana* eggs. Saline wet preparation of faeces. [38] Lower magnification, [39] higher magnification. Note the two shells, the presence of characteristic polar filaments (arrow) between the two layers, and three pairs of hooklets in the embryo.

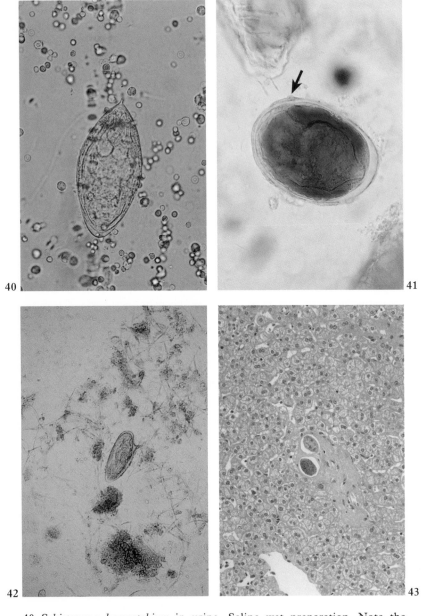

40 *Schistosoma haematobium* in urine. Saline wet preparation. Note the characteristic terminal spine on the egg.

41 *Schistosoma japonicum* egg in faeces. Saline wet preparation. Note the characteristic small lateral spine on the egg.

42 *Schistosoma mansoni* egg in faeces. Saline wet preparation. Note the characteristic large lateral spine on the egg.

43 Granuloma in liver around the egg of *Schistosoma* spp. (*S. mansoni or S. japonicum*) in a case of hepatic schistosomiasis. The rest of the architecture of the liver is preserved. H & E stain.

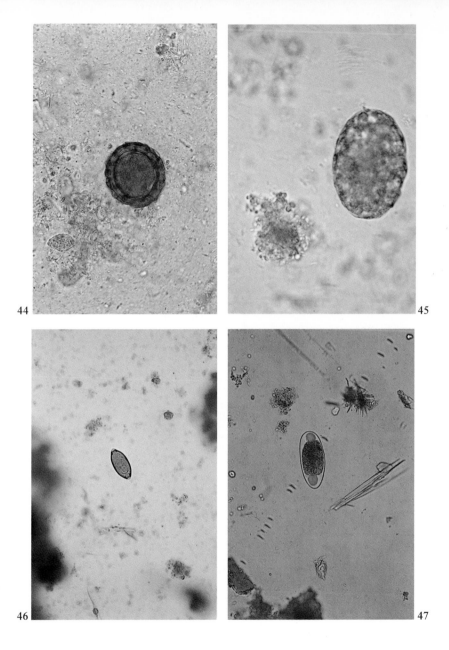

44, 45 *Ascaris lumbricoides* eggs in faeces. Saline wet preparation. [44] Fertilised eggs. [45] Unfertilised eggs. The yellow-brown, mamillated external layer (corticated) shown here, is characteristic. Decorticated fertile eggs may also be seen.

46 *Trichuris trichiura* egg in faeces. Saline wet preparation. Note that the 'tea-tray' appearance (with polar plugs) is similar to *Trichostrongylus* spp. eggs.

47 *Trichostrongylus* spp. egg in faeces. Saline wet preparation.

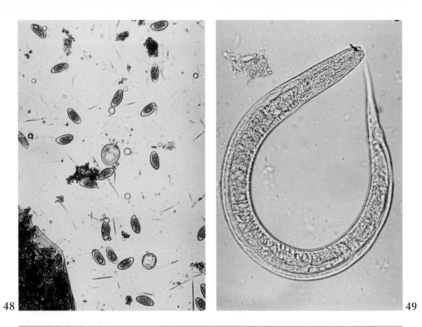

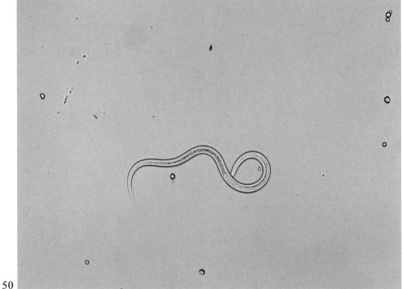

48 *Enterobius vermicularis* eggs expelled from a gravid female worm. Saline wet preparation. The eggs have a characteristic plano-convex shape (football shape with one side flattened).

49, 50 *Strongyloides stercoralis* in faeces. Saline wet preparations. [49] Rhabditiform larva with a shorter buccal cavity (arrow) differentiates it from hookworm larvae; [50] filariform larva (from Harada culture). Eggs are not seen in *S. stercoralis* infection.

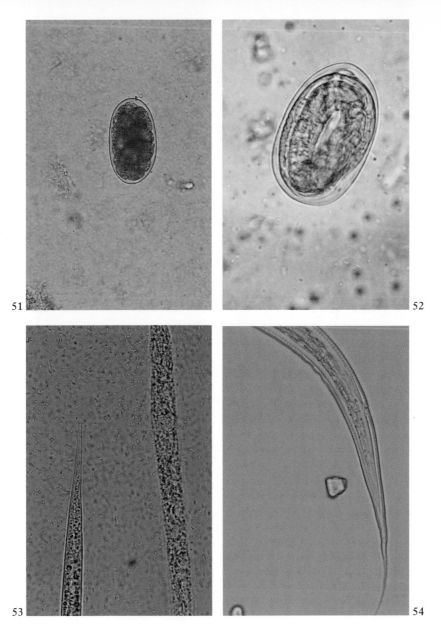

51, 52 Hookworm in faeces. Saline wet preparations. [51] Egg, which has a thin
outer layer and a multi-lobed embryo (usually 4–16 lobes). [52] Egg with a
larva about to hatch. This stage is seen when the faecal specimen has been
standing at room temperature for some time.

53, 54 Close-up of filariform larvae of [53] *Strongyloides*, which has a notched
tail, and [54] hookworm, which has a tapering tail.

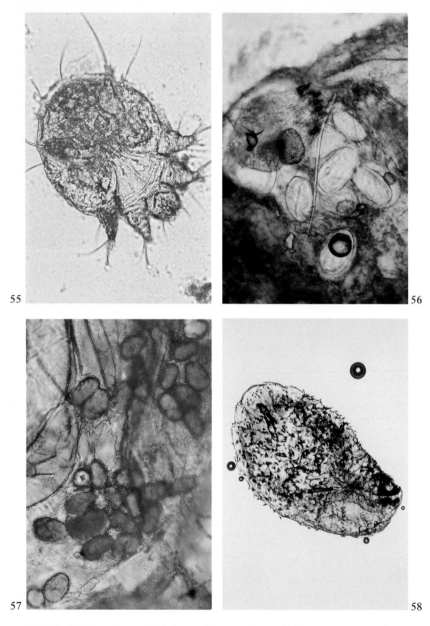

55, 56, 57 *Sarcoptes scabei* from skin scrapings. Saline wet preparations. [55] Adult mite, [56] eggs and larva, [57] faecal pellets.

58 Maggot (larval form) of botfly (*Dermatobium hominis*) from a swelling on the thigh of a traveller returned from Africa.

TREATMENT

Patients should be hospitalised for treatment.[74,75] Cases in returned travellers are presumed choloroquine-resistant unless infection was unequivocally obtained in a chloroquine-sensitive area. Quinine resistance appears to be increasing, especially in Thailand, but is still uncommon in returned travellers.

Oral treatment:

Quinine sulfate
Children: 10 mg salt/kg three times a day (max. 600 mg)
Adults: 600 mg three times a day

Parenteral treatment (if sick or high parasitaemia):

Quinine dihydrochloride
Loading dose: 20 mg salt/kg iv in 500 mL of 5% glucose by rate-controlled infusion over 4 hours
Maintenance: 10 mg salt/kg iv over 4 hours, 8 hourly until oral therapy is tolerated. Commence 4 hours after loading dose is completed.

Both oral and parenteral quinine should be combined with:

Doxycycline* 100 mg twice daily for 7 days, or once daily for 10 days, commenced while the patient is in hospital

or **Pyrimethamine–sulfadoxine** 3 tabs on last day of quinine therapy (for areas where resistance is limited).

If quinine resistance is suspected:[17,76]

Artesunate 100 mg iv twice daily in oily solution for 2 doses followed by 50 mg twice daily for 8 doses (total 600 mg over 5 days)

or **Atovaquone + proguanil** (Malarone)
Children
11–20 kg: 1 tab (250 mg/100 mg) stat for 3 consecutive days
21–30 kg: 2 tabs stat for 3 consecutive days
31–40 kg: 3 tabs stat for 3 consecutive days
Adults
>40 kg: 4 tabs stat for 3 consecutive days

Mefloquine and **halofantrine** are alternatives to quinine and artesunate therapy but halofantrine is associated with cardiac toxicity and is not generally recommended.[17]

> * Do **not** use doxycycline in pregnant women or children aged 8 years or less.
>
> Quinine is **not** given with mefloquine; avoid a loading dose if the patient has been taking mefloquine or quinine prophylaxis.
>
> The bisulfate salt of quinine has only 70% of the activity of the sulfate salt and appropriate dosage adjustments should be made.[4]

Exchange transfusion may be required for high parasitaemia ($\geq$ 10–15%).

FOLLOW UP

Monitor the clinical course; manage the anaemia, hypoglycaemia, pulmonary oedema and renal failure as they occur. Repeat T+T blood smears until there are no detectable parasites and again 2–4 weeks after therapy to detect recurrences due to drug-resistant parasites.

Plasmodium vivax, P. ovale and *P. malariae*

CLINICAL NOTES

Symptoms and signs are usually indistinguishable from those of *P. falciparum*. Fever is more likely to be periodic, occurring every 48 hours with *P. vivax* and *P. ovale*, and every 72 hours with *P. malariae*. Serious complications are not usually a feature of malaria caused by these species because sequestration of parasitised erythrocytes does not occur. Relapsing *P. vivax* and *P. ovale* infections may present 2–5 years after exposure, but usually occur in the first 6 months. Recurrent *P. malariae* infection may be seen 30–40 years after leaving endemic areas. *P. malariae* has been associated with the nephrotic syndrome.

> **Suspect malaria in any traveller with fever returning from an endemic area.**

DIAGNOSIS

- Examine T+T blood smears for parasites as for *P. falciparum* (see Plates 25–27).
- Screen for G6PD deficiency before treatment with primaquine.

- A rapid diagnostic antigen test has recently been introduced for *P. vivax* (AMRAD-ICT Malaria P.f/P.v).[73]
- PCR and serology are available in special circumstances as for *P. falciparum.*

TREATMENT

Chloroquine phosphate   (300 mg base = 2 tablets salt)

Children: 10 mg of base/kg (max. 600 mg of base) po, then 5 mg of base/kg in 6 hours, and on days 2 and 3

Adults: 600 mg base stat po, 300 mg po 6 hours later and 300 mg po on days 2 and 3

> Chloroquine-resistant *P. vivax* has been reported in PNG, Indonesia and elsewhere. If this is suspected, treatment with quinine should be commenced (see *P. falciparum*).

Radical cure for relapses in *P. vivax* or *P. ovale* (following chloroquine therapy):

Primaquine phosphate*
Children: 0.3 mg of base/kg once a day po for 14 days (a liquid preparation can be prepared by pharmacy)
Adults: 15 mg of base daily, orally with food for 14 days or 45 mg of base once a week for 8 weeks

> * Primaquine is contraindicated in pregnancy.
>
> Relapses may recur after primaquine treatment.
>
> For *P. vivax* malaria acquired in the Pacific, use primaquine 15 mg twice daily or 7.5 mg three times a day.

FOLLOW UP

Monitor T+T blood smears until there are no detectable parasites and again if symptoms recur.

PROPHYLAXIS

The risk of developing malaria ranges from 7–9 per 1000 travellers in PNG and the Solomons to 4 per 100 000 travellers in Malaysia. It is important to educate travellers about minimisation of exposure to mosquito bites as well as to prescribe chemoprophylaxis where appropriate.[74,75]

Chemoprophylaxis in adult travellers:

The need for and type of chemoprophylaxis will depend on the anticipated duration and intensity of exposure to malaria, as well as the pattern of drug resistance in the areas of travel.

- Areas with chloroquine-sensitive malaria

    Chloroquine   300 mg base/week (usually 2 tablets).

- Areas with chloroquine-resistant malaria

    Doxycycline★   100 mg/day commenced 1 day before and then taken during travel and for 4 weeks after leaving the malaria endemic area

or   **Mefloquine★**   250 mg/week commenced 1 week before and then taken weekly during travel and for 4 weeks after leaving the malaria endemic area.

- Areas with mefloquine-resistant malaria

    Doxycycline★   100 mg/day

★ Mefloquine is **not** used in children less than 15 kg body weight, and should be avoided in the first trimester of pregnancy and in lactating females. WHO recommends that the drug may be given with confidence during the second and third trimesters of pregnancy.

For women in the first trimester of pregnancy who cannot postpone travel to an area where there is a high prevalence of chloroquine-resistant malaria, consider using chloroquine and proguanil.

Mefloquine is contraindicated in those with a history of epilepsy or psychiatric disorder, and in those involved in tasks requiring fine co-ordination and spatial discrimination.

Quinine may be used as standby treatment in an emergency.

★ Do **not** use doxycycline in pregnant women or in children aged 8 years or less.

The chloroquine dose in children is 5 mg/kg per week up to the maximum adult dose.

For those living in endemic areas for long periods, consider using no prophylaxis or chloroquine in urban (low prevalence) areas and adding doxycyline for short trips to rural (higher prevalence) areas.

> Chloroquine and proguanil (200 mg daily) may be more effective than chloroquine alone in some areas and may be considered in those in whom mefloquine and doxycycline are contraindicated.
>
> Standby treatment regimes (quinine or Malarone) may be useful in some cases, but are seldom prescribed by the authors.

DRUG AVAILABILITY IN AUSTRALIA

Artesunate not currently available in Australia, but may be imported for use in exceptional circumstances
Atovaquone–Proguanil
    Malarone: 250 mg Atovaquone + 100 mg Proguanil
Chloroquine   *Chlorquin:* 50 mg (= 155 mg base) tabs
Doxycycline   *Doryx:* 50 mg, 100 mg caps
              Vibramycin: 50 mg, 100 mg tabs
Halofantrine [SAS approval]
    Halfan: 50 mg tabs or 100 mg/5 mL suspension
Mefloquine   *Lariam:* 250 mg tabs
Primaquine [SAS approval]   7.5 mg, 15 mg base tabs
Pyrimethamine-sulfadoxine   *Fansidar:* 25 mg, 500 mg tabs
Quinine dihydrochloride [SAS approval]
Quinine sulfate   *Quinate:* 300 mg tabs

Pneumocystis carinii

A fungus, when classified on genetic analysis of several chromosomal and mitochondrial genes, but morphologically and biologically similar to a protozoan

LIFE CYCLE AND EPIDEMIOLOGY

The life cycle is still incompletely understood. There are three morphologically distinct stages: a trophozoite stage, where the organisms probably multiply by binary fission; a cyst stage, with mature cysts (5–8 μm) containing 6–8 intracystic bodies; and pre-cystic stages, which are intermediate between trophozoites and cysts.

There is a worldwide distribution and *P. carinii* is found in the environment as well as in the lungs of healthy humans and animals. Indeed, about 60% of the population are sero-positive. Symptomatic infections appear to be due to reinfection rather than reactivation. Risk factors include HIV infection, anti-cancer chemotherapy, immunosuppression associated with organ transplantation or vasculitis, and hypogammaglobulinaemia.

CLINICAL NOTES

The most common presentation is pneumonia. The predominant symptoms are dyspnoea, non-productive cough and fever of days to weeks duration (may be longer in patients with AIDS). Auscultation is usually normal or there may be fine basal crepitations or wheeze. Haemoptysis and pleuritic chest pain are unusual. If the infection is untreated, symptoms worsen over days to weeks and the patient usually dies. Extrapulmonary lesions occur in a minority (< 3%) of patients. The lymph nodes, spleen, liver and bone marrow are most frequently involved.

DIAGNOSIS

- Demonstration of *P. carinii* cysts or trophozoites in broncho-pulmonary secretions obtained as induced sputum or BAL material. Special stains are used, including immunofluorescence (IF), toluidine blue (see Plate 2) and methenamine silver. IF is probably the most sensitive test available routinely, and is preferred by many laboratories. Microscopy of induced sputum is usually sufficient to make the diagnosis in HIV-infected patients (sensitivity when compared to bronchoscopy varies from 50 to 90%), but in non-

HIV-infected patients, BAL and/or open lung biopsy may be necessary. Bronchoscopy may, however, be useful to make a definitive diagnosis of other causes of pneumonia in HIV-infected patients.[77]

- CXR shows bilateral diffuse infiltrates in advanced cases. In early disease the chest may appear normal or show a perihilar haze only. Atypical X-ray appearances occur, including unilateral consolidation, nodules, cavities and pleural effusions.
- Impaired oxygenation is usual even with a normal CXR.

TREATMENT

Primary treatment:

Trimethoprim-sulfamethoxazole[4,78]

TMP (15–20 mg/kg per day) + SMX (75–100 mg/kg per day) po (i.e. 8 DS tablets/day) or iv, in 3 or 4 doses for 21 days.

Neutropenia, anaemia, rash, fever are common.

Alternative treatments:

Pentamidine 3–4 mg/kg per day (max. 300 mg) iv in 50–250 mL of 5% glucose infused during 1 hour, for 21 days. Nephrotoxicity, leucopoenia, hypotension, and hypoglycaemia are common.

or **Dapsone** 100 mg/day for 21 days, *and*

Trimethoprim 15–20 mg/kg per day in 4 divided doses for 21 days.

Corticosteroids should also be used in moderate to severe cases.

In patients unable to tolerate these drugs, **clindamycin** and **primaquine** in combination or **atovaquone** may be used.[17]

Prophylaxis and maintenance therapy (if CD4 < 0.25×10^9/L):

Trimethoprim-sulfamethoxazole 1 DS tablet once or twice daily three times a week (i.e. Mon, Wed and Fri)

or **Dapsone** 100 mg po three times a week

or **Pentamidine** 3–4 mg/kg per day (max. 300 mg) iv every 2–4 weeks or 300 mg via nebuliser monthly

or **Dapsone** 100 mg po twice a week, *and*

Trimethoprim 300 mg po twice a week.

Test patient for G6PD deficiency if dapsone or primaquine is used.

FOLLOW UP

Monitor the clinical course carefully as patients may continue to deteriorate in the first few days after commencement of therapy. The CXR may not improve for 7–10 days. Adverse reactions to TMP-SMX and pentamidine occur in up to 80–90% of patients. If the reaction is mild (fever and rash), therapy may be continued. Desensitisation may be attempted in certain cases.[4]

DRUG AVAILABILITY IN AUSTRALIA

Atovaquone [SAS approval] *Mepron:* 250 mg tabs
Dapsone *Dapsone 100:* 100 mg tabs
Pentamidine *Pentamidine isethionate for injection* BP: 300 mg vials
Trimethoprim *Triprim:* 300 mg tabs
Trimethoprim-sulfamethoxazole
  Bactrim or *Septrin* or *Resprim:* 80 mg, 400 mg tabs
  Bactrim DS or *Septrin Forte* or *Resprim Forte:* 160 mg, 800 mg tabs
  Co-trimoxazole solution BP: 80 mg trimethoprim + 400 mg sulfamethoxazole/5 mg ampoules

Sarcoptes scabei

Arachnida: itch mite, mange mite

LIFE CYCLE AND EPIDEMIOLOGY

Scabies is highly contagious. Transmission is through person-to-person contact either with direct skin or with fomites. *Sarcoptes scabei* undergoes four stages in its life cycle: egg, larva, nymph and adult. Adult female mites form burrows under the skin in which eggs are deposited every 2–3 days and which incubate in 3–8 days. After the eggs hatch, the mites migrate to the skin surface and moult. There is a higher incidence in institutionalised people, especially the aged, and mentally compromised or immunocompromised persons. Scabies occurs worldwide.

Animal scabies occurs in mammals such as domestic cats, dogs, pigs and horses, but these species do not establish infestations in humans. However, the mites may cause self-limited pruritis in humans due to dermatitis.

CLINICAL NOTES

Scabies presents with severe pruritis associated with erythematous papules and excoriations, especially in the interdigital web spaces, wrists, elbows, anterior axillary folds, periumbilical skin, pelvic girdle, penis, knees and ankles. Persons who have had a previous infestation may develop symptoms within a few days due to prior sensitisation to the mite. Classical **linear burrows** are only occasionally present and may be difficult to find. Secondary bacterial infection is common in children.

'Norwegian' or crusted scabies occurs in immunocompromised patients (especially associated with corticosteroid use and AIDS). In this condition there are numerous mites, but only slight itching. The clinical features include widespread hyperkeratotic crusted nodules and plaques. Burrowing does not occur. Septicaemia may result from secondary bacterial infection. Norwegian scabies is highly infectious.

DIAGNOSIS

- Clinical history of severe pruritis and the appearance and distribution of the rash, and the presence of burrows (may not be present).
- Microscopic examination of skin scrapings for the presence of adult mites, larval stages, eggs or faecal pellets. Scrapings over a

burrow are taken with a scalpel or sharp needle to the depth of pinpoint bleeding and sent to the laboratory as soon as possible. A positive microscopy result is dependent on the load of adult mites (numerous in Norwegian scabies) and the quality of scraping (see Plates 55–57).

TREATMENT

Permethrin 5% Massage from head to soles of feet. Wash after 8–12 hours. Repeat 1 week later if moderate or severe infection. Safe in children aged 2 months and older. Resistance has been reported.[79]

or **25% benzyl benzoate** or **10% crotamiton** Apply as directed.

Norwegian scabies:

Permethrin should be applied after a hot bath and again 12 hours later (and leave on for 12 hours). Repeat after 1 week.

Alternatively, use **ivermectin*** 200 µg/kg single dose po.[80]

> Ivermectin should be used WITH CAUTION for treatment of scabies in elderly patients because of increased toxicity.

Systemic **antibiotics** (especially anti-*Staphylococcus*) may be necessary to treat local infections and avoid sepsis.

FOLLOW UP

For eradication, it is important to treat close contacts (even if symptomless). Clothes and bed linen should be washed in hot water. Monitor the clinical course and if required repeat the skin scrapings. Pruritis may continue for weeks after successful treatment. A mild steroid cream may be required in sensitive individuals.

DRUG AVAILABILITY IN AUSTRALIA

Benzyl benzoate *Ascabiol* 25% emulsion
Crotamiton *Eurax* 10% cream/lotion
Ivermectin *Stromectol:* 6 mg tabs
Permethrin 5% *Lyclear* 5% cream
                   Quellada 5% lotion

Schistosoma spp.

Trematodes: blood flukes

LIFE CYCLE

Human schistosomiasis is caused by three main species: *Schistosoma haematobium*, *S. mansoni* and *S. japonicum* (*S. intercalatum* and *S. mekongi* are less common). Infection is acquired when swimming or bathing in fresh water in endemic areas. After penetration of the skin, the cercariae are carried to the liver where they mature into adult worms and the males and females pair off. Worm pairs migrate to the superior and inferior mesenteric veins (*S. mansoni* and *S. japonicum*, respectively) or pelvic veins (*S. haematobium*) where they produce eggs from 4 to 12 weeks after exposure until they die 3–8 years later. The eggs are moved progressively toward the lumen of the intestine (*S. mansoni* and *S. japonicum*) and of the bladder and ureters (*S. haematobium*), and are passed with faeces or urine, respectively. The eggs hatch and release miracidia, which then infect the snail intermediate host within 8–12 hours (for this reason schistosomes are sometimes called 'snail worms'). Production of the infective larvae (i.e. cercariae) occurs in 1–2 months. Ectopic schistosome eggs are sometimes found in the CNS with all species, but particularly with *S. japonicum*.

Schistosomiasis is second only to malaria as a major parasitic cause of morbidity and mortality in developing countries. The prevalence of schistosomiasis in travellers returning from endemic areas has also increased in recent years. In a recent study the prevalence of undiagnosed asymptomatic schistosomiasis in travellers exposed to fresh water in Zimbabwe, Botswana or Malawi was 9%.[82]

Schistosoma haematobium

EPIDEMIOLOGY

Schistosoma haematobium is confined to Africa and the Middle East.

CLINICAL NOTES

Cercarial dermatitis (swimmer's itch) occasionally occurs within 24 hours of cercarial penetration. Acute schistosomiasis (Katayama fever) is rare (see *S. japonicum*).

Schistosoma haematobium infection produces granulomatous reactions and fibrosis in the bladder. Early, light infections may be asymptomatic in returned travellers. The most common complaint is recurrent painless **haematuria**. Dysuria, urinary frequency and suprapubic pain also occur. It is important to exclude coexistent bacteriuria. In chronic infection the inflammatory response to eggs leads to marked fibrosis. Patients present with urinary obstruction, hydronephrosis, pyelonephritis and renal failure. **Bladder cancer** is a rare, late presentation that is thought to be associated with urinary schistosomiasis. Rarely, there may be involvement of the male genital organs, especially the prostate, leading to discoloured ejaculate and infertility.[83] Recurrent *Salmonella* bacteraemia is a recognised complication.

> In Australia, cercarial dermatitis more commonly occurs on exposure to avian schistosomal cercariae and symptoms are more intense than with the human strains.

DIAGNOSIS

- Microscopic examination of terminal urine (best collected between noon and 2 p.m.) for eggs is the main method of diagnosis. Occasionally ectopic eggs are found in faeces. In difficult cases microscopic examination of bladder or rectal tissue may yield a positive result. Eggs are sometimes seen in semen.[83] Schistosomes are speciated according to the appearance of the eggs. Eggs become apparent in urine 5–13 weeks after infection, but as they may be passed intermittently or in small amounts, their detection will be enhanced by repeated examinations and centrifugation and examination of the sediment (see Plate 40).
- Estimation of the number of eggs is possible by filtration of a standard volume of urine through a Nucleopore membrane followed by egg counts on the membrane.

> Most returned travellers have a low worm burden and no detectable eggs, so the diagnosis is made by serology.

- **Serology** An IHA assay using *S. mansoni* antigen from adult flukes is commonly used. Serology may be negative in early infections, but antibodies can generally be detected prior to eggs being found in faeces. Assay is genus specific with sensitivities of approximately 95% or more for *S. mansoni*, 90% for *S. haematobium* and 50% for *S. japonicum* and *S. mekongi*.[84] Mean titres are low for species other than *S. mansoni*. Antibody levels may remain elevated for several months or years after successful treatment. False negative results are generally due to early infections, so monitoring of patients for

6–12 months after exposure is recommended. False positive results may occur in patients with other parasitic infections and those who have been infected with avian schistosomes. An EIA test that uses egg antigens and has similar sensitivity and specificity is also available. Species-specific testing is performed at CDC, Atlanta.

• Peripheral eosinophilia may be present.

TREATMENT

Praziquantel 20 mg/kg twice daily orally for 1 day.

This is sufficient for treatment in field programs, but some centres now use 20 mg/kg twice daily for 3 days for the treatment of individual patients, especially if symptomatic, because of concern about treatment failure with praziquantel.[85–88]

Minor side effects with praziquantel are common and include malaise, headaches, dizziness, nausea and vomiting.

FOLLOW UP

Urine or faecal microscopy to show disappearance of eggs 1 month after therapy. For patients without detectable eggs, serology performed 6–12 months after treatment may show a falling titre (although high titres may persist for a few years).

Schistosoma intercalatum

EPIDEMIOLOGY

This infection is not a serious public health problem in endemic areas and is rare in tourists. There is a very limited geographic distribution with endemic foci described in Chad, Cameroon, Congo, Zaire, Gabon and the Central African Republic.

CLINICAL NOTES

Schistosoma intercalatum may cause **intestinal** or **urinary schistosomiasis**. Symptoms are usually mild or absent. Children and adolescents may present with abdominal pain and diarrhoea. Haematuria has also been reported.

DIAGNOSIS

• Microscopic examination of faeces and/or multiple rectal snips (via proctoscope) for eggs, and also examination of terminal urine (collected between noon and 2 p.m.) for ectopic eggs. Speciation is according to the appearance of the eggs.

- The sensitivities and specificities of the currently available serological tests for *S. intercalatum* are not well defined.
- Peripheral eosinophilia may be present.

TREATMENT

Praziquantel 20 mg/kg twice daily po for 1 day.

FOLLOW UP

Repeat microscopy to show disappearance of eggs 1 month after therapy.

Schistosoma japonicum

EPIDEMIOLOGY

There are endemic foci in China, including a major focus in southern China along the Yangtze River basin. The infection is also endemic in the Philippines and central Sulawesi.

CLINICAL NOTES

Cercarial dermatitis may occur within 24 hours of cercarial penetration.

Katayama fever (acute schistosomiasis) is most common in *S. japonicum* infection and may occur 2–10 weeks after infection. Features include fever, headache, cough, abdominal pain, diarrhoea, hepatosplenomegaly, lymphadenopathy and urticaria. Cerebral and spinal cord involvement may occur. Katayama fever is most marked in primary infections in non-immune individuals. The illness usually resolves in a few weeks, but may be fatal.

Intestinal schistosomiasis develops later and, although many patients will be asymptomatic, some present with fatigue, abdominal pain and chronic diarrhoea. In chronic *S. japonicum* infections with moderate to heavy worm burden, portal hypertension, hepatosplenomegaly, oesophageal varices, and ascites may occur. Hepatocellular failure with hepatic encephalopathy does not develop unless there is coexistent hepatitis B or C virus infection. Pulmonary hypertension may occur with both *S. mansoni* and *S. japonicum*.

Cerebral schistosomiasis presenting as epilepsy or a space-occupying lesion is an important clinical difference between *S. japonicum* and the other species.

DIAGNOSIS

- Microscopic examination of faeces and/or multiple rectal snips (via proctoscope) for eggs, and also examination of terminal urine (collected between noon and 2 p.m.) for ectopic eggs. Speciation is according to the appearance of eggs (see Plate 41).
- **Serology** IHA and EIA have a lower sensitivity for *S. japonicum* than the other species, but may be positive in approximately 50% of cases. In suspected cases in which eggs are undetectable, confirmatory testing should be considered (see *S. haematobium* for more details).
- A CT scan with or without biopsy is indicated if CNS disease is suspected.
- Peripheral eosinophilia occurs and is pronounced in Katayama fever.

TREATMENT

Praziquantel 30 mg/kg twice daily po for 1 day.

FOLLOW UP

Repeat faecal microscopy to confirm disappearance of eggs 1 month after therapy. Repeat serology after 6–12 months (although high titres may persist for years).

Schistosoma mansoni

EPIDEMIOLOGY

Schistosoma mansoni infection is endemic in many Africa countries, Saudi Arabia, Brazil, Surinam, Venezuela and the West Indies.

CLINICAL NOTES

As with the other species, **cercarial dermatitis** occurs occasionally. **Katayama fever** is uncommon, but may be increasing due to poor control measures in some countries.

Continuing infection produces granulomatous reactions and fibrosis and the manifestations of **intestinal schistosomiasis**. This may vary from asymptomatic to severe depending on duration and worm burden. Most patients are asymptomatic, but those with heavy infection have chronic or intermittent bloody diarrhoea, fatigue, anorexia, abdominal pain, weight loss and fever. Later, portal hypertension, hepatosplenomegaly, oesophageal varices, and ascites may occur. Hepatocellular failure is usually associated with coexistent hepatitis B or C infection. Pulmonary hypertension may occur with both *S. mansoni* and *S. japonicum.*

Spinal cord schistosomiasis is more common in *S. mansoni* than the other species and may occur in the acute stage or during established infection.

DIAGNOSIS

*   Microscopic examination of faeces and/or multiple rectal snips (via proctoscope) for eggs and also examination of terminal urine (collected between noon and 2 p.m.) for ectopic eggs. Speciation depends on the appearance of eggs (see Plates 42, 43).

> Most returned travellers have a low worm burden and no detectable eggs, so the diagnosis is made by serology.

*   **Serology** (See *S. haematobium* for details). Mean serum titres of persons suffering from *S. mansoni* are between 1:256 and 1:1024. Sensitivity is 95% or more.
*   Peripheral eosinophilia may occur (especially in Katayama fever).

TREATMENT

Praziquantel 20 mg/kg twice daily po for 1 day.

This is sufficient for treatment in field programs, but some centres now use 20 mg/kg twice daily for 3 days for the treatment of individual patients, especially if symptomatic, because of concern about treatment failures with praziquantel.[85–88]

Oxamniquine is an alternative in selected patients.[33]

FOLLOW UP

Repeat microscopy to confirm disappearance of eggs 1 month after therapy. For patients without detectable eggs, serology performed 6–12 months after treatment may show a falling titre (although high titres may persist for a few years).

Schistosoma mekongi

EPIDEMIOLOGY

Infection is geographically confined to and thought to be the main human species in mainland Indo-China (Mekong River basin: Cambodia, Laos and Vietnam).

CLINICAL NOTES

Clinical features are similar to *S. japonicum* infection, but milder. In one study of Laotian patients, hepatomegaly was the most prominent finding. Cerebral and cardiopulmonary complications have not been reported. Morbidity may be compounded by other parasitic infections in the same area, such as *Opisthorchis viverrini*.

DIAGNOSIS

• Microscopic examination of faeces and/or multiple rectal snips (via proctoscope) for eggs and also examination of terminal urine (collected between noon and 2 p.m.) for ectopic eggs. *Schistosoma mekongi* eggs are smaller than those of *S. japonicum*.
• The sensitivities and specificities of the currently available serological tests for *S. mekongi* are not well defined.
• Peripheral eosinophilia may occur.

TREATMENT

Praziquantel 30 mg/kg twice daily po for 1 day.[89]

FOLLOW UP

Repeat microscopy to show disappearance of eggs 1 month after therapy.

DRUG AVAILABILITY IN AUSTRALIA

Oxamniquine **[SAS approval]** *Vansil* (Contact Pfizer for direct importation.)
Praziquantel *Biltricide:* 600 mg tabs

Spirometra spp.

Cestodes: larval cyst (sparganum) is found in humans

Dogs and cats are the usual definitive host for this tapeworm. Eggs are excreted in faeces, hatch in fresh water, and then the larvae are ingested by and undergo the first stage of development in the water flea (copepods). When the second intermediate host (fish, reptiles, frogs and other animals such as chickens) ingests the copepods, a tissue larval cyst (sparganum) develops. The sparganum develops into an adult tapeworm upon ingestion by a dog or cat, thus completing the life cycle.

Human infection (sparganosis) is acquired by ingestion of raw or undercooked poultry, frogs and snakes and also by the application of frog or snake-meat poultices to wounds or inflamed eyes. As well, infection can be acquired by drinking water that contains infected copepods. The sparganum (a small, white, ribbon-like worm) causes an inflammatory response as it migrates through tissues. Human infections are caused by several species including *S. mansoni*, *S. mansonoides* and *S. theilleri*.

The infection is endemic in East Africa, South East Asia, China, Japan and South America. It is rarely reported in Europe, North America and Australia.[90]

CLINICAL NOTES

Sparganosis is an uncommon human infection that presents as inflamed subcutaneous swellings and nodules, usually on the chest or legs. The nodules can be migratory. **Ocular sparganosis** manifests as pruritis, pain, lacrimation and swelling of the eyelids. Involvement of other tissues, including the CNS, has also been described.[90] The disease should be differentiated from gnathostomiasis and loiasis. A rare proliferative form of the infection exists, which slowly progresses to death (aberrant spargana).

DIAGNOSIS

- Surgical removal and microscopic identification of the worm. Spargana do not have suckers or hooklets and so can be differentiated from a cysticercus.
- Serological testing is not currently available in Australia.
- Eosinophilia and leucocytosis are common.

TREATMENT

Surgical removal of the spargana is the recommended treatment.

There is **no effective drug treatment**, although surgical treatment along with praziquantel did produce resolution of a nodule and eosinophilia in one case.[90]

FOLLOW UP

Monitor the clinical course.

Strongyloides stercoralis

Intestinal nematode

LIFE CYCLE AND EPIDEMIOLOGY

Transmission is by contact with soil or surface water containing filariform larvae, which enter through intact skin and travel to the lungs where they penetrate the alveolar spaces and are carried through the bronchial tree to the pharynx. They are then swallowed and reach the intestine where they mature to adult worms. Eggs hatch within the bowel and the resulting rhabditiform larvae pass out in the faeces approximately 1 month after infection and become either infectious (filariform larvae) or free-living adult males and females, which mate and produce rhabditiform larvae. The latter in turn can either develop into new free-living adults, or into infective filariform larvae. In some patients rhabditiform larvae become infectious within the bowel and can reinvade enteric mucosa or perianal skin to cause a build up in the number of adult worms in the intestine. This process is called 'autoinfection' and the filariform larvae usually follow the previously described route (i.e. via the lungs, the bronchial tree, the pharynx, to the small intestine). Autoinfection can sometimes be maintained for decades.

The infection occurs widely in the tropics and subtropics and less commonly in temperate areas. There is a high prevalence in South East Asia, Brazil and Colombia. The infection is more common in those living in rural areas, institutions and in lower socio-economic groups.

CLINICAL NOTES

Approximately 30% of infected individuals are asymptomatic, maintaining infection with a small number of worms by autoinfection. A history of 'ground itch', or pruritic rash at the site of larval penetration may be elicited.

Pulmonary symptoms (Loeffler-like syndrome) and eosinophilia may occur as the larvae penetrate the alveolar spaces.

Intestinal symptoms include intermittent watery diarrhoea, nausea, vomiting, abdominal pain and weight loss. Malabsorption may occur.

A cutaneous linear eruption (**larva currens**) is associated with migration of larvae under the skin. Urticarial skin rashes on the buttocks and around the waist also occur in individuals who have become sensitised to larval antigens.

Chronic strongyloidiasis may be complicated by secondary Gram-negative septicaemia or meningitis.

In immunocompromised patients, autoinfection may lead to massive larval invasion of the lungs and intestines (**hyperinfection syndrome** or 'disseminated strongyloidiasis'). Patients can present with abdominal pain, distension, shock, pulmonary and neurological complications and septicaemia. The prognosis is poor.

DIAGNOSIS

- Peripheral eosinophilia is usually present (but may be intermittent) during the acute and chronic stages and is especially associated with autoinfection and pulmonary symptoms, but may be absent with dissemination.
- Microscopic examination of faeces, duodenal fluid (from an Entero-Test or duodenal aspiration) and/or sputum for worms, rhabditiform larvae or eggs (see Plates 49, 50). Faecal microscopy is relatively insensitive and so multiple specimens and concentrates should be examined (sensitivity > 80% if 4–5 concentrated specimens examined).
- Harada culture of faeces to detect filariform larvae also increases sensitivity.
- **Serology** An EIA using soluble antigens from third-stage *Strongyloides ratti* larvae is available. It does not distinguish current from past infections although there is evidence that antibody levels decline slowly after successful treatment (1–2 years in some cases). The sensitivity and specificity are 93% and 95%, respectively (State Health Laboratories, Perth, WA, Australia). Others report sensitivities of 80–92% and specificities of 90–94%.[91] There is cross-reactivity with sera from patients with filarial and other nematode infections.

TREATMENT

Albendazole 400 mg twice daily po for 3 days

or **Ivermectin** 200 µg/kg per day single dose po for 1–2 days (especially in immunocompromised patients)

or **Thiabendazole** 25 mg/kg twice daily po (max. 3 g/day) for 3 days (not used commonly because of unpleasant side effects)

Repeat after 7 days if complications are present. The treatment is not always successful, especially in immunocompromised patients. Repeat at monthly intervals or give longer courses in these patients.

FOLLOW UP

Repeat faecal examination 1 month after therapy.

DRUG AVAILABILITY IN AUSTRALIA

Albendazole   *Eskazole:* 400 mg tabs
                     Zentel: 200 mg tabs
Ivermectin   *Stromectol:* 6 mg tabs
Thiabendazole   *Mintezol:* 500 mg tabs

Taenia spp.

Cestodes: tapeworms

Taenia saginata (beef tapeworm)

LIFE CYCLE AND EPIDEMIOLOGY

Humans are the only definitive host, and cattle are the intermediate hosts for *T. saginata*. Humans acquire the infection by ingesting undercooked beef containing infective larval cysts (cysticerci). In the human intestine, the cysticercus develops in 2–3 months into an adult tapeworm, which grows up to 25 metres in length and can survive for more than 30 years. Worms are made of numerous proglottids, which become gravid and detach from the tapeworm and are passed in the stool. The eggs contained in the gravid proglottids (80 000–100 000 eggs per proglottid) are released after the proglottid becomes free and has been passed with the faeces. The eggs can survive for months to years in the environment. Humans may harbour more than one worm, each of which sheds proglottids containing eggs in the faeces.

Cattle acquire the infection when their feed or grazing pasture is contaminated with eggs or proglottids. The oncosphere is released from the egg in the animal intestine and migrates to striated muscle where it develops into a cysticercus that may survive for several years.

The highest prevalence (more than 10%) is in cattle in middle and western South Asia and Central and East Africa.

CLINICAL NOTES

The infection is usually asymptomatic or produces mild abdominal cramps and malaise. Proglottids are motile and may be felt emerging from the anus or found on the perineum or clothing or seen in faeces. Rarely, appendicitis or cholangitis can result from migrating proglottids.

DIAGNOSIS

- Demonstration of *T. saginata* eggs (indistinguishable from *T. solium*) or proglottids in the faeces. Repeated examination and concentration techniques will increase the likelihood of detecting light infections. Eggs will not be apparent in faeces for the first 3 months after infection (see Plates 34, 35).
- To distinguish *T. saginata* from *T. solium*, examine the proglottids after injecting dye (such as India ink) and count the number of

uterine branches (*T. saginata* has 15–20 lateral branches). There is some overlap between the species and other morphological features may be needed for certain identification. Other techniques such as staining the whole proglottid, serial sectioning to study the anatomy of the genital pore or using DNA probes have been described, but are not routinely available.

TREATMENT

Praziquantel 10–20 mg/kg stat po

or **Niclosamide** 2 g stat chewed.

Treatment kills the adult worm only, *not* eggs.

FOLLOW UP

Repeat faecal examination for eggs or proglottids 1–3 months after therapy.

Taenia solium (pork tapeworm)

LIFE CYCLE AND EPIDEMIOLOGY

The life cycle of *T. solium* is similar to that of *T. saginata*. Humans are one of the definitive hosts (also monkeys and hamsters), and pigs are the intermediate hosts. Human taeniasis is acquired by ingestion of raw or undercooked pork containing infectious larval forms (cysticerci). Adult worms develop from these cysticerci in the intestine and grow to 8 metres and survive for up to 20 years. Humans can also be infected by ingesting *T. solium* eggs passed by a human carrier (different from *T. saginata*) either in food contaminated with faeces, or by autoinfection. Oncospheres that develop from the eggs may lead to human cysticercosis (see later section).

Endemic areas include South East Asia, India, Philippines, southern Europe, Africa, Mexico, and Central and South America. The infection is more prevalent in poorer communities where humans live in close contact with pigs and eat undercooked pork. It is rare in the Muslim population.

CLINICAL NOTES

Taeniasis Most carriers of adult *T. solium* worms are unaware of their infection. As with *T. saginata*, mild gastrointestinal symptoms do occur, but the main symptom is often the passage (passive) of proglottids. The main concern is that carriers and household members are at risk of acquiring cysticercosis by the faecal–oral route.

DIAGNOSIS

- Demonstration of *T. solium* eggs (indistinguishable from *T. saginata*) or proglottids in the faeces. Repeated examination and concentration techniques will increase the likelihood of detecting light infections. Eggs will not be apparent in faeces for the first 3 months after infection (see Plates 34, 35).
- To distinguish *T. solium* from *T. saginata*, examine the proglottids after injecting dye (such as India ink) and count the number of uterine branches (*T. solium* has 7–13 lateral branches).

Extreme care is needed when processing the samples.
Ingestion of eggs can result in cysticercosis.

TREATMENT

> **Praziquantel** 5–10 mg/kg stat po

or **Niclosamide** 2 g stat chewed.

Treatment kills the adult worm only, *not* eggs.

FOLLOW UP

Repeat faecal examination for eggs or proglottids 1–3 months after therapy.

Cysticercosis (larval form of *T. solium*)

LIFE CYCLE

Human cysticercosis is acquired by ingesting *T. solium* eggs that have been shed by a human tapeworm carrier. Infection may be acquired by faecal–oral autoinfection. Autoinfection occurs when a human infected with a *T. solium* tapeworm ingests eggs produced by that tapeworm, either through faecal contamination or, perhaps, from proglottids carried into the stomach by reverse peristalsis. Ingested taenia eggs develop into invasive larvae (oncospheres) in the small intestine. These migrate across the intestinal wall and are carried in the blood to the sites in which they will mature into cysticerci (≈ 2 months). The cysticercus develops not only in striated muscle, but also in the brain, liver and other tissues of humans as well as in pigs and other animals.

Cysticercosis is increasingly diagnosed in developed countries due to the long life of the worm in human carriers who may have been born in, or travelled in, endemic areas and are unaware of their infection.

CLINICAL NOTES

The commonest clinical manifestation of **neurocysticercosis** is late onset epilepsy[92]. Other symptoms and signs are so varied that diagnosis may be difficult. All parts of the CNS may be affected and pathology includes intracerebral lesions (causing mass effect or epilepsy), intraventricular cysts (causing hydrocephalus), sub-arachnoid lesions (causing chronic meningitis with lymphocytic or eosinophilic pleocytosis), spinal cord lesions (causing cord compression leading to progressive paraplegia) and cisternal cysticercosis. Cysts enlarge slowly over years and the onset of symptoms often correlates with cyst death. Cerebral ischaemia, subacute encephalitis and brain stem syndromes also occur.

Subcutaneous nodules (cysts) are common in some areas of the world, occurring in 6–79% of individuals with neurocysticercosis. They usually produce few symptoms and eventually calcify as do the nodules that may also occur in the skeletal muscles, eye and heart.

Ocular cysticercosis is uncommon and usually presents as a scotoma.

Racemose cysticercosis is a rare aberrant form of *T. solium* in which clusters of interconnected cysts with no identifiable proto-scolex are detected in the brain (usually in the cisternal magna or ventricles). Surgery is the mainstay of therapy.

DIAGNOSIS

- Radiological imaging is usually required to make a diagnosis. CT and MRI show multiple enhancing and non-enhancing unilocular cysts (see Plate 37). Calcified lesions are common. However, a negative scan does not exclude the diagnosis.
- Histological examination of biopsy material (subcutaneous nodules or brain tissue) and the demonstration of the larvae (see Plate 36).
- Peripheral and/or CSF eosinophilia is common.
- **Serology** An EIA using cyst vesicular antigen to detect antibodies (primarily IgG) to *T. solium* is available. There is significant cross-reactivity with other diseases, including *Echinococcus*-positive samples (up to 50%), filariasis and *T. saginata*. Antibody response is influenced by cyst location. There is lower sensitivity in neurocysticercosis patients with a single enhancing or calcified parenchymal cyst. Test sensitivity is higher for serum samples (≈ 80% in most studies) than CSF samples. A positive test result should therefore be investigated by immunoblot (sensitivity 98%, specificity 100%), and by CT or MRI.

TREATMENT

Corticosteroids (e.g. dexamethasone) should be used along with anticysticercal therapy because degenerating cysticerci can induce a marked inflammatory response, which may be fatal.

and **Albendazole** 15 mg/kg per day in 3 doses for 8–15 days

or **Praziquantel** 20 mg/kg three times daily for 14 days

It is important to start the steroids first.

Dexamethasone has been shown to decrease praziquantel levels and to increase albendazole levels, but this seems to be of little clinical significance.

The use of anticysticercal drugs is controversial as some trials show little benefit over symptomatic treatment.[92,93] They should **not** be given during the acute phase of severe cysticercotic encephalitis. Nor are they required for calcified cysts. Treatment should be individualised in each patient based on the location and viability of cysts, symptoms and the degree of host inflammatory response.

Albendazole appears more efficacious than praziquantel, but the drugs may be used together in refractory cases.

Minor side effects with praziquantel are common.

The dose of praziquantel may need to be increased when antiepileptics and corticosteroids are used concurrently.

In ocular cysticercosis, use albendazole cautiously and avoid praziquantel.

Surgical resection and/or **ventricular shunting** are usually reserved for hydrocephalus and ventricular and spinal cysts.

Antiepileptic therapy should be used as necessary.

FOLLOW UP

Monitor clinically and radiologically:
* response to therapy, and
* progress of the cyst if anticysticercal drugs have not been given.

DRUG AVAILABILITY IN AUSTRALIA

Albendazole *Eskazole:* 400 mg tabs
              Zentel: 200 mg tabs
Niclosamide *Yomesan:* not currently available in Australia
Praziquantel *Biltricide:* 600 mg tabs

Toxocara canis, Toxocara cati

Tissue nematodes: ascarid species of dogs and cats

Toxocara canis and *T. cati* cause roundworm infection in dogs and cats, respectively, and humans are accidental hosts. In *T. canis* infection, eggs are passed in canine faeces (mainly puppies and lactating bitches) and mature in 3–4 weeks. Humans acquire the infection by ingestion of embryonated eggs in contaminated soil. Eggs hatch in the stomach, and larvae enter the mesenteric vasculature and are distributed to the liver, and in some cases, throughout the body. The larvae do not undergo any further development, but may provoke a granulomatous reaction. Children playing in contaminated soil are particularly at risk. There is a worldwide distribution.

CLINICAL NOTES

Often larvae are quickly destroyed by the host immune response without causing any symptoms. There are two main clinical presentations.

Visceral larva migrans (VLM) is most common in young children, who present with fever, hepatomegaly, cough and wheezing (pneumonitis), and eosinophilia due to invasion of multiple tissues by larvae. Urticaria, nodules, nephritis and CNS manifestations also occur. Death can occur rarely, by severe cardiac, pulmonary or neurological involvement. Most cases are self-limiting. VLM should be differentiated from ascariasis and strongyloidiasis. Other animal ascarid larvae also cause VLM.

Ocular larva migrans (OLM) occurs when a larva becomes entrapped in the eye. This results in an eosinophilic inflammatory mass that later causes an area of retinal degeneration. Low-grade iridocyclitis may be present. Vision may be impaired if the lesion is central. Usually there are no systemic symptoms or signs and eosinophilia is rare. The disease is more common in older children or young adults and should be differentiated from retinoblastoma and ocular toxoplasmosis.

DIAGNOSIS

- A presumptive diagnosis of VLM or OLM is based on clinical signs, history of exposure to puppies, laboratory findings (including eosinophilia), and the detection of antibodies to *Toxocara*.

- Eosinophilia is pronounced in children with VLM, but rare in OLM.
- **Serology** An EIA using *T. canis* third-stage larval excretory–secretory antigens is available. The sensitivity has been reported as 78% in patients with VLM, but is less in those with OLM. There is cross-reactivity with strongyloidiasis, filariasis and fascioliasis, which may not be relevant unless the geographic area includes a high prevalence of these infections. Antibody levels remain elevated for years. The ability of this assay to differentiate *T. canis* from *T. cati* infection is unknown.
- Histopathological detection of larva in affected tissues may occasionally be possible.
- Fluorescein angiography, ultrasound or CT scan may be useful in OLM.

TREATMENT

Treat only if clinical disease is present.[32]

Visceral larval migrans:

Diethylcarbamazine 2 mg/kg three times daily for 10 days

or **Albendazole** 400 mg twice daily for 3–5 days (≈ 50% effective).

Ocular larval migrans:

There is no specific therapy for OLM, so treat with **corticosteroids** (local or intraocular) followed by DEC (as for VLM). **Laser photocoagulation** may be useful.[94]

FOLLOW UP

Monitor the clinical course. Prevention is by regular treatment of dogs and puppies for roundworms.

DRUG AVAILABILITY IN AUSTRALIA

Albendazole *Eskazole:* 400 mg tabs
 Zentel: 200 mg tabs
Diethylcarbamazine *Hetrazan:* 50 mg tabs

Toxoplasma gondii

Tissue protozoan

LIFE CYCLE AND EPIDEMIOLOGY

Felines (members of the cat family) are the definitive hosts. When infected, they excrete large numbers of oocysts in faeces for a 1–2 week period, which then form infectious sporocysts in 3–4 days. Sporocysts are very resistant and may remain infectious in the soil for up to 1 year. Intermediate hosts (often farm animals) become infected by grazing on contaminated pastures. Human infection is acquired by ingestion (or handling) of tissue cysts in raw or poorly cooked meat (especially lamb and pork), or other food contaminated with oocysts, or from contact with faeces from infected cats (especially kittens). Congenital transmission may occur if there is primary maternal infection just before or during pregnancy. Toxoplasmosis is rarely acquired from an organ transplant, blood transfusion or laboratory accident. The parasites form tissue cysts, most commonly in skeletal muscle, myocardium and brain; these cysts may remain viable throughout the life of the individual. Immunodeficient patients are at risk of developing reactivated disease.

There is a worldwide distribution, and seroprevalences range from 22 to 85% in different communities and age groups. Infection is more common in warm climates and at lower altitudes.

CLINICAL NOTES

Congenital toxoplasmosis The incidence and severity of congenital toxoplasmosis depend on the trimester during which infection was acquired, being more severe in the first and second trimesters. Manifestations include spontaneous abortion, chorioretinitis, hydrocephalus, epilepsy and mental retardation. Most infants with subclinical infection at birth will develop signs or symptoms of congenital toxoplasmosis during the next 20 years of life unless the infection is treated. Ocular toxoplasmosis is usually a result of congenital infection and patients may be asymptomatic until the second or third decade of life, when lesions develop in the eye. Treatment of the mother reduces the incidence of congenital infection, so early diagnosis is important.

Acquired toxoplasmosis

Immunocompetent patients The incubation period is 2–3 weeks. Most individuals are asymptomatic, but the infection may persist as tissue cysts for many years. However, 10–20% of patients with acute infection develop painless cervical lymphadenopathy sometimes with fever and malaise. The illness is benign and self-limited (symptoms may last for a few months to 1 year) and should be differentiated from lymphoma, tuberculosis and infectious mononucleosis.

Immunocompromised patients Reactivated infections may occur in the CNS (encephalitis, space-occupying lesion) or, less commonly, in other organs (chorioretinitis, pneumonitis and myocarditis). In patients with AIDS, toxoplasmic encephalitis is the most common cause of intracerebral mass lesions and is usually due to reactivation of latent infection. Toxoplasmosis in patients being treated with immunosuppressive drugs may be due to either newly acquired or reactivated latent infection. Occasionally, primary infections may occur in heart transplant recipients and in AIDS patients in areas where transmission of toxoplasma is high.

DIAGNOSIS

- Histology or touch preparations of cells or tissues (e.g. brain, lymph node, heart, lung aspirate or biopsy) for identification of tachyzoites or tissue cysts, with or without specific staining (see Plates 3, 4).
- Isolation of toxoplasma from selected samples, which must be transported to the laboratory as soon as practicable. Tachyzoites are relatively labile. This test may not always be available.
- Toxoplasma DNA detection by PCR. This test is available at VIDRL, Melbourne, and CIDM, Westmead Hospital, Sydney, at the level of experimental assessment.
- **Serology** is the primary method of diagnosis (even though the prevalence of antibodies in Australia is 30–50%). Tests available include EIA and IFA for IgG and IgM to tachyzoites. IgG antibodies persist indefinitely. A single high level is not diagnostic of recent or active infection. A significant rise between two samples is defined as a four-fold rise in titre by IFA and a two-fold rise by EIA. IgM antibodies by EIA frequently persist for more than 1 year. IgM antibodies by IFA seldom persist for more than a few weeks or months.

Seroconversion of IgG and detection of IgM confirm acute infection in an **immunocompetent host**.

In the **immunocompromised patient** with reactivated infection, a significant rise in IgG may occur (e.g. those with AIDS, or organ or bone marrow transplants). Reactivated ocular infection is usually not associated with a rise in antibodies.

In **pregnant women** with serology suggestive of a recent infection (seroconversion, high IgM and clinical suspicion) further investigation is necessary. The most effective method for diagnosing fetal infection is to test amniotic fluid and fetal blood for toxoplasma DNA by PCR and specific anti-toxoplasma IgM, as well as to attempt toxoplasma isolation by cell culture and animal inoculation. Ultrasound may also show fetal abnormalities. After delivery, detailed clinical examination of the neonate should be combined with PCR, serology and toxoplasma isolation. Specific, high-titre neonatal IgM (positive in 75%, but may develop postnatally) or persistent IgG after the disappearance of maternal IgG are highly suggestive of neonatal infection. The sensitivity of a PCR assay using amniotic fluid has been reported as 97.4% and the negative predictive value as 99.7% in one study.[95]

TREATMENT

Pyrimethamine 100 mg twice daily po on the first day, then 25–50 mg/day for 2–4 weeks in immunocompetent patients, or 4–6 weeks in immunocompromised patients (maintenance dose in AIDS is 25 mg/day), given with 7.5 mg of **folinic acid** in orange juice,

with **Sulfadiazine** loading dose of 75 mg/kg (up to 4 g) po or iv then 2–4 g/day (maintenance dose in AIDS is 500 mg four times daily)

or with **Clindamycin** 300–600 mg four times daily po for 3–6 weeks

or with **Azithromycin** loading dose 1750 mg po then 1250 mg daily for 3–6 weeks (maintenance dose in AIDS is 500 mg/day).

Higher doses of all drugs may be required in the acute stages in AIDS.[96]

Corticosteroids may be required in ocular and CNS disease.

Maintenance dose is given lifelong.

Atovaquone (750 mg four times daily) may be useful in refractory cases.

Maternal infections:

Spiramycin 1 g three times daily.

FOLLOW UP

Monitor the clinical course and radiology.

DRUG AVAILABILITY IN AUSTRALIA

Pyrimethamine   *Daraprim:* 25 mg tabs

Sulfadiazine   *Sulphadiazine* injection BP: 4 mL vials (1 g/4 mL)

Clindamycin   *Dalacin C:* 150 mg caps; 600 mg/4 mL ampoules; 75 mg/5 mL syrup

Folinic acid   *Leucovorin calcium:* 15 mg tabs

Azithromycin   *Zithromax:* 250 mg, 500 mg, 600 mg tabs; powder for oral suspension 200 mg/5 mL

Spiramycin [SAS approval]

Rovamycin: 500 mg caps; 1.5 MIU/ampoule (Contact Aventis for direct importation.)

Trichinella pseudospiralis
Trichinella spiralis

Tissue nematodes

Humans are not the normal host for *Trichinella* spp. and infection is only acquired by the ingestion of tissue cysts in poorly cooked, contaminated meat (usually pork sausage in the classic form of trichinosis caused by *T. spiralis*). After ingestion, larvae are released, attach to intestinal villi and develop into adult worms. Female adults produce larvae that seed into skeletal muscles (and occasionally the brain and heart) via the blood stream. Larvae encyst (except for *T. pseudospiralis*) in 17–21 days and may remain viable for years or eventually calcify. In the Americas and in Europe *T. spiralis* is usually an infection of rats, which are ingested by domestic pigs.

Trichinella spp. are found in virtually all warm-blooded animals and the incidence has increased with the eating of exotic wild game (e.g. wild boar, walrus and cougar jerky).[97] *Trichinella pseudospiralis* is found in animals and birds worldwide including marsupials in Australia, especially in Tasmania. An outbreak of *T. pseudospiralis* following consumption of raw pork was reported in 1998.[98] Subspecies include *T. s. nativa* (Arctic bears), *T. s. nelsoni* (African predators and scavengers) and *T. s. bitovi* (carnivores of Europe and western Asia). Small foci of disease have been reported in Africa (due to *T. s. nelsoni*) and the Arctic due to the ingestion of undercooked bear meat (*T. s. nativa*).

CLINICAL NOTES

Trichinosis is a self-limiting infection lasting weeks to months. Light infections are often asymptomatic. Heavy exposure may lead to nausea, vomiting and diarrhoea during the intestinal stage, and periorbital and facial oedema, conjunctivitis, fever, myalgia, splinter haemorrhages, rashes and blood eosinophilia during the tissue migration stage (1 week after infection). Skin rashes and pneumonitis usually occur in the first week; myalgia, weakness, periorbital oedema, headache, and fever occur in the second and third weeks. In severe cases, myocarditis, meningoencephalitis with a variety of focal deficits, and ocular disturbances may occur. In these cases the brain shows multiple ischaemic areas throughout the pons and white matter. In the final stage of encystment, there may be cachexia, oedema and dehydration. However, in most patients, symptoms begin to resolve during the second month. Chronic symptoms have been reported. It is important to differentiate trichinosis from the acute stages of other tissue-invasive helminth infections as well as from connective tissue diseases. Vertical transmission to the fetus has been described.[99]

DIAGNOSIS

- Demonstration of coiled larvae by microscopy in muscle biopsy tissue.
- **Serology** An EIA is available using excretory–secretory antigen purified from *T. spiralis* larvae. The test becomes positive 3–5 weeks post-infection. Acutely ill patients present early and are thus likely to be serologically negative. Eventually 80–100% of symptomatic patients will have positive serology. False negative results occur in lightly infected individuals. The specificity is excellent. Titres fall significantly in 1–2 years.
- Hyper-eosinophilia is usual from the 14th day.
- Muscle creatine phosphokinase and lactate dehydrogenase may be elevated.
- Radiology may show calcified cysts.

TREATMENT

The mainstay of therapy is **bed rest** with:

Salicylates 300–600 mg three times daily

and/or **Corticosteroids** 20–60 mg/day po for 3–5 days, then taper

plus **Mebendazole** 200–400 mg three times daily for 3 days then 400–500 mg three times daily for 10 days

or **Albendazole** 400 mg for 3 days.

> Albendazole and mebendazole are active against the intestinal stages, but not the encysted larvae. Corticosteroids decrease the severity of symptoms during the muscle invasion phase.

FOLLOW UP

Monitor the clinical course, eosinophil count and serology.

DRUG AVAILABILITY IN AUSTRALIA

Albendazole *Eskazole:* 400 mg tabs
Zentel: 200 mg tabs
Mebendazole *Banworm:* 100 mg tabs
Sqworm: 100 mg tabs
Vermox: 100 mg tabs; 100 mg/5 mL suspension

Trichomonas vaginalis

Flagellate protozoan

Trichomonas vaginalis is non-invasive, usually existing free in the vagina or attached to the epithelium. In males, the urethra is often involved and only rarely are the epididymis and prostate. The parasite does not appear to have a cyst form, and does not survive well outside the genital tract. The disease is primarily an STD of humans. Vertical transmission to female neonates during passage through the birth canal also occurs. There is a worldwide distribution.

CLINICAL NOTES

The incubation period is 5–28 days. Female patients usually present with vaginal discharge (malodorous, irritating, greenish-yellow, frothy). Symptoms may also include dyspareunia, dysuria and lower abdominal pain. An asymptomatic carrier state also exists, but is unusual. In men, infection is usually asymptomatic and self-limiting. Urethritis, epididymitis and prostatitis can occur. There is no evidence of serious consequences although *T. vaginalis* has been reported as a rare cause of neonatal pneumonia.[100]

DIAGNOSIS

• Accurate diagnosis depends on demonstrating the organism in genital specimens.[100] Trophozoites with characteristic motility may be observed in wet mount preparations of vaginal secretions in 50–80% of infected women, and in preparations from an anterior urethral swab in 50–90% of men. Ensure the specimen is fresh and not contaminated with faecal material (non-pathogenic *T. hominis* is found in the GIT and has similar morphology).
• Direct immunofluorescent antibody staining is more sensitive than wet mount preparations, but is technically more difficult.
• Culture on trichomonas medium (modified Diamond's medium is the best) has a sensitivity of > 95%.
• It is important to exclude coexisting STDs.

TREATMENT

Metronidazole★ 2 g stat po or 250 mg three times daily for 7 days

or **Tinidazole★** 2 g stat po

> ★ Metronidazole and tinidazole should be avoided in the first trimester of pregnancy, or if lactating, interrupt breast feeding for 24 hours.

In pregnancy:

> **Clotrimazole** 100 mg vaginal pessary at bedtime for 1–2 weeks *then* later in pregnancy or after delivery give **metronidazole** (as above).

> Metronidazole resistance is reported and higher doses may be required. Alternative drugs such as **furazolidone** and **mebendazole** have been shown to be effective.

FOLLOW UP

Monitor the clinical course. Treat sexual partners, even if asymptomatic.

DRUG AVAILABILITY IN AUSTRALIA

Clotrimazole *Canesten* vaginal: 100 mg vaginal tabs
Metronidazole
    Flagyl: 200 mg, 400 mg tabs; 200 mg/5 mL suspension
    Metrogyl: 200 mg, 400 mg tabs; 200 mg/5 mL suspension
Tinidazole *Fasigyn:* 500 mg tabs
               Simplotan: 500 mg tabs

Trichostrongylus spp.

Intestinal nematodes

LIFE CYCLE AND EPIDEMIOLOGY

Trichostrongylus nematodes primarily infect sheep and goats, but occasionally infect humans. These small worms are similar to hookworms and live in the intestinal mucosa. Human infection is acquired orally through the ingestion of contaminated plant material or through the skin. Maturation occurs in the intestine in 3–4 weeks without a pulmonary migration phase. The eggs are passed in faeces and hatch in a warm moist environment (i.e. soil) and become infective in 2–3 days.

There is a higher incidence in people living near the grazing areas of herbivores. Infection is widespread in Africa, Asia, Indonesia and Japan.

CLINICAL NOTES

The infection is asymptomatic in most cases as the worm burden is light. However, there may be a history of pruritic rash at the penetration site. If the worm burden is high, patients may present with gastrointestinal symptoms in the early phase (abdominal pain, diarrhoea, weight loss) and later develop iron-deficiency anaemia and chronic malnutrition (especially in children).

DIAGNOSIS

- Microscopic demonstration of eggs in faecal specimens. *Trichostrongylus* eggs are similar to, and sometimes confused with, hookworm eggs (see Plate 47).
- Eosinophilia may occur.

TREATMENT

Albendazole   400 mg stat po

or   **Pyrantel embonate**   10 mg/kg stat (max. 750 mg).

FOLLOW UP

Repeat faecal examination 2–4 weeks after therapy.

DRUG AVAILABILITY IN AUSTRALIA

Albendazole   *Eskazole:* 400 mg tabs
              Zentel: 200 mg tabs

Pyrantel embonate   *Anthel:* 125 mg, 250 mg tabs
                    Combantrin: 125 mg, 250 mg tabs
                    Early Bird: 100 mg chocolate squares

Trichuris trichiura

Intestinal nematode: whipworm

LIFE CYCLE AND EPIDEMIOLOGY

Transmission of *Trichuris trichiura* is by ingestion of eggs from soil-contaminated hands or food. The eggs then hatch in the small intestine and release larvae that mature. The adult worms attach firmly in the appendix, caecum and ascending colon. The unembryonated eggs appear in faeces about 2 months after infection. In the soil they embryonate and become infective in 15–30 days. The life span of adult worms is about 1 year.

The infection is most prevalent in children (5–15 years), and estimates suggest that 800 million individuals may be infected worldwide, especially in warm, moist areas with poor sanitation. *Trichuris trichiura* is often found together with *Ascaris lumbricoides*.

CLINICAL NOTES

Patients are usually asymptomatic or have mild abdominal discomfort. In heavily infected individuals there may be epigastric pain, vomiting, anorexia and weight loss (especially if associated with another parasite). Some patients develop dysentery with bloody diarrhoea, and rectal prolapse. In severe chronic cases anaemia and growth retardation have been reported. It is important to differentiate this infection from hookworm infection and amoebic dysentery, both of which also cause blood loss and anaemia.

DIAGNOSIS

- Microscopic demonstration of eggs in faecal specimens. Concentration techniques improve the yield (see Plate 46).
- Adult worms can occasionally be found by examining the rectal mucosa by proctoscopy (or directly in the case of a prolapse).

TREATMENT

Mebendazole
≤ 10 kg: 50 mg twice daily po for 3 days
> 10 kg: 100 mg twice daily po for 3 days

or **Albendazole**
≤ 10 kg: 200 mg stat po
> 10 kg: 400 mg stat po

FOLLOW UP

Repeat the faecal examination 2–4 weeks after therapy. A second course may be required to eradicate the infection.

Trichuris trichiura

Albendazole   *Eskazole:* 400 mg tabs
                 Zentel: 200 mg tabs
Mebendazole *Banworm:* 100 mg tabs
                 Sqworm: 100 mg tabs
                 Vermox: 100 mg tabs; 100 mg/5 mL suspension

Trypanosoma spp.

Protozoa: haemoflagellates

Trypanosoma brucei (*gambiense* and *rhodesiense*)

LIFE CYCLE AND EPIDEMIOLOGY

West African trypanosomiasis is caused by *T. b. gambiense*. Transmission is by tsetse flies (*Glossina palpalis* group) and is most intense in forests and wooded areas along rivers. The infection is therefore primarily a problem in rural populations. The parasites mature and multiply in the fly and are then inoculated when the fly bites another mammal. Trypanosomes multiply in the host's blood and extracellular fluids such as spinal fluid. Humans are the main reservoir for *T. b. gambiense*, but this subspecies can also be found in animals. The infection occurs in Central and West Africa.

East African trypanosomiasis is caused by *T. b. rhodesiense*. Transmission is also by tsetse flies (*Glossina morsitans* group), which are widely distributed in savanna and woodlands in East and South Africa. Cattle and wild animals serve as the main reservoir. Epidemics occur. Tourists to game parks are occasionally infected.

CLINICAL NOTES

Sleeping sickness has a varied presentation. Early on there is a local nodule or a chancre at the site of inoculation (only occurs in *T. b. rhodesiense* and may last for several weeks). This is followed by the haemolymphatic stage: symptoms include intermittent fever, headaches, malaise, rash, anaemia, oedema, lymphadenopathy and hepatosplenomegaly. The meningoencephalitic stage is progressive with late manifestations of mood changes, daytime somnolence, mental deterioration, coma and death.

East African trypanosomiasis produces a rapid, fulminating disease with high parasitaemia and severe early symptoms 2–3 weeks post-infection. Death may occur in a few months, before CNS involvement develops. In tourists, fever, malaise and headache may appear before the end of the trip or shortly after returning home.

West African trypanosomiasis is characterised by lower parasitaemia, less severe initial manifestations and chronic progression of disease. Untreated patients may survive for years.

DIAGNOSIS

- Demonstration of trypanosomes on microscopic examination of wet preparations and Giemsa-stained smears of chancre fluid, lymph node aspirates (multiple samples if there is a high index of suspicion), bone marrow aspirates and T+T blood films. It is important to examine multiple samples and use concentration techniques, as parasite numbers may be low.

- Examine CSF to determine the stage of the disease: CNS involvement if trypanosomes are present and/or leucocytes are ≥ 5 cells/mL and/or there is elevated protein.
- An elevated serum IgM and ESR (high negative predictive value if normal) is supportive evidence of the diagnosis.
- **Serology** An IHA to detect antibodies to purified *T. b. gambiense* antigen is available. (The humoral immune response with the East African form is poor, making serodiagnosis of little value.) Non-specific reactions are common and organisms should be identified for definite diagnosis. Negative serology with concomitant parasitaemia may occur, especially in the early stages of the disease. The Card Agglutination Trypanosomiasis Test (CATT) is of value for epidemiological surveys or screening of *T. b. gambiense*.

Care must be taken in the laboratory, as trypomastigotes are highly infectious.

TREATMENT

Early disease:

> **Suramin** 200 mg iv (test dose), then 1 g iv on days 1, 3, 7, 14 and 21

or **Pentamidine** 3–4 mg/kg (base) im per day or alternate days for 10 days (not effective in *T. b. rhodesiense*).

Late disease:

> **Melarsoprol** given iv very slowly (extremely toxic) increasing the dose over 30 days (total of 1300 mg)[17]

> **Eflornithine (DFMO)** has recently been shown to be effective in early and late *T. b. gambiense* infection.[101]

FOLLOW UP

Early disease:
Repeat T+T blood smears 1–2 months after therapy.

Late disease:
Monitor CSF analysis during and after therapy. It may be necessary to follow patients for up to 2 years.

Trypanosoma cruzi

LIFE CYCLE AND EPIDEMIOLOGY

Trypanosoma cruzi infection is a zoonosis transmitted by reduviid bugs, which are widely distributed in the wild and also live in and around substandard dwellings. Feeding on human or animal blood that contains circulating parasites infects the reduviid bugs. The parasites are then released in the insect faeces near the site of the bite during a subsequent blood meal. Infection occurs through breaks in the skin, mucous membranes or conjunctivae. In humans, trypanosomes transform into intracellular amastigotes that mature in a variety of cells and multiply and release trypomastigotes into the circulation. These trypomastigotes do not replicate, but replication resumes when the parasites enter another cell and transform into amastigotes. Trypomastigotes are ingested by the reduviid bug as it obtains a blood meal.

Trypanosoma cruzi can also be transmitted through blood transfusion, transplacentally, and in laboratory accidents. Dogs and domestic animals are important reservoirs. The infection occurs all over Latin America. It is rare in returned travellers.

CLINICAL NOTES

Acute **Chagas' disease** is usually an illness of children. An erythematous swelling at the site of entry of the parasite ('chagoma'), or painless oedema of the palpebrae and periocular tissues (Romana's sign) may occur at the site of inoculation. Fever, malaise, oedema, lymphadenopathy, and hepatosplenomegaly and myocarditis sometimes follow. This acute illness usually resolves over a few months.

Chronic Chagas' disease may then appear years later with cardiomyopathy (usually at 30–40 years of age), arrhythmias, cerebral embolism, mega-oesophagus or megacolon. The mega-syndromes are rare, but may occur in young patients. Reactivation of infection may occur as a result of immune dysfunction (including HIV infection). Chronic Chagas' disease and its complications can be fatal.

DIAGNOSIS

- In acute disease, microscopic examination of T+T blood films, buffy coats, lymph node aspirate, bone marrow aspirate, CSF and pericardial fluid for parasites (positive in > 90% of cases).
- Xenodiagnosis (where uninfected reduviid bugs are fed on the patient's blood, and their gut contents are examined for parasites 4 weeks later) and culture on special media such as NNN or LIT may be available in some centres.

- Lymphocytosis and an abnormal ECG are common.
- **Serology** The most important method for the diagnosis of chronic disease. An IFA is available that detects antibodies to trypomastigotes of *T. cruzi*. Sensitivity is approximately 90%, although negative results occur in both early and late disease. Specificity is lower as cross-reactivity with sera from patients with malaria, syphilis, leishmaniasis and lepromatous leprosy occurs. A positive test should be confirmed by a different serological method. Conflicting results are common. A fourfold or greater rise in titre between acute and convalescent sera indicates active acute phase disease. A fourfold or greater decrease indicates a convalescent phase. Titres normally decrease significantly within the first year after successful treatment, and after 2 years more than 80% of cases have negative serology. In chronic disease, serology remains positive for life, but may be detected only by the newer very sensitive techniques.

TREATMENT

Current therapy is unsatisfactory. However, two drugs are being used.

Nifurtimox
Children 1–10 years: 15–20 mg/kg in 4 doses for 90 days
          11–16 years: 12.5–15 mg/kg in 4 doses for 90 days
Adults   10 mg/kg in 3 doses for 90–120 days

or   **Benzidazole** 5–10 mg/kg po for 30–60 days.

- Only 50% cure rate in chronic cases. Higher rates of cure may be seen if treated in the early chronic phase.[102]
- Acute Chagas' disease must be treated early and the decision to treat should be made on clinical and epidemiological grounds while awaiting laboratory confirmation.

Surgery may be required in the chronic disease.

FOLLOW UP

Repeat T+T blood smears or xenodiagnosis 1–2 months after therapy. Monitor serology and ECG.

DRUG AVAILABILITY IN AUSTRALIA

Benzidazole **[SAS approval]** *Rochagan:* not currently available in Australia. Contact Roche for direct importation.

Eflornithine (DFMO) [SAS approval]
Ornidyl: not currently available in Australia. Contact Aventis for direct importation.

Melarsoprol [SAS approval] *Arsobal:* not currently available in Australia. Contact Aventis for direct importation.

Nifurtimox [SAS approval] *Lampit:* not currently available in Australia. Contact Bayer for direct importation.

Pentamidine *Pentamidine isethionate for injection* BP: 300 mg vials

Suramin [SAS approval] not currently available in Australia. Contact Bayer for direct importation.

Wuchereria bancrofti and *Brugia* spp.

Filarial nematodes

These parasites are transmitted by female mosquitoes. Adult worms (up to 100 mm in length) may reside in the lymphatics and lymph nodes of the human host for several years. The female worms produce microfilariae that appear in the blood after 3–8 months (depending on species) and may then be ingested by the vector. Microfilariae appear in the blood with differing periodicity, depending on the biting habits of the local vector.

Wuchereria bancrofti occurs widely in the tropics; *Brugia malayi* is confined to East and South East Asia and South India; *B. timori* is restricted to eastern Indonesia. It is unusual for tourists to become infected unless there has been intense exposure for many months. Complications develop only after repeated inflammatory attacks. Filariasis is occasionally diagnosed in migrants from endemic areas.

CLINICAL NOTES

Clinical manifestations may vary depending on the species and geographical location. The manifestations are dominated by the patient's immune response. Microfilaraemia occurs in the presence of immune unresponsiveness and only in a proportion of cases. A summary of common manifestations is included below.

Bancroftian and Brugian filariasis Many patients are asymptomatic despite the presence of microfilaraemia. Symptomatic patients usually have acute episodes of fever (filarial fevers), tender lymphadenopathy, lymphangitis and swollen legs (or oedema elsewhere). Episodes may occur several times a year and last for 3–7 days. Many cases do not have microfilaraemia, and inflammation may be evoked by a host response to worm antigens. Epididymitis, orchitis and chronic lymphadenopathy and hydrocoele (*W. bancrofti*) are reported. Abscesses may form along the lymphatic system or at the lymph node. Eventually the effects of chronic lymphatic obstruction, including elephantiasis of the limbs and scrotum and chyluria, may become evident. Ulceration and secondary bacterial infection often occurs. Monoarticular arthritis may occur.

Tropical pulmonary eosinophilia This syndrome presents with dry nocturnal cough and occasional haemoptysis, wheezing, fever and marked eosinophilia. Symptoms often occur at night. CXR shows diffuse miliary lesions. There is marked eosinophilia, but usually no circulating microfilariae. The symptoms are probably due to hyperreactivity to filarial antigens in the lungs, and microfilariae may be found in lung biopsy specimens.

DIAGNOSIS

- Demonstration of microfilariae in peripheral blood samples collected at midnight (except for infections acquired in the Pacific region, in which case parasites are maximal between noon and 8 p.m.). The blood sample may be examined as a wet, or microhaematocrit, preparation, and T+T smears including buffy coat smears. Sensitivity is increased by concentration techniques such as the Knott technique in which the blood is lysed in 2% formalin or by filtration through a membrane. In some cases a DEC provocation test may increase the yield of microfilariae in the blood. Patients may be amicrofilaraemic in early and late disease.
- **Serology** An EIA using heterologous antigens from the adult worm of the dog filarial species *Dirofilaria immitis* is available to detect circulating antibodies (see *Loa loa* for further details of the EIA antibody test).
- Antigen detection using a rapid immunochromatographic test is available (from Amrad-ICT Diagnostics, Australia). This assay specifically recognises *W. bancrofti* antigen in human blood and is both sensitive and specific. Cross-reactions do not occur with other human filarial infections or gastrointestinal helminths. A negative test virtually excludes ongoing infection.
- Molecular diagnosis using PCR is available for *W. bancrofti* and *B. malayi* in some laboratories.
- Imaging of lymphatics may be of use in amicrofilaraemic cases.
- Eosinophilia is common during episodes of acute inflammation.

TREATMENT

Diethylcarbamazine
Day 1: 50 mg po, after food
Day 2: 50 mg three times daily
Day 3: 100 mg three times daily
Days 4–21: 6 mg/kg per day in 3 doses

or **Ivermectin** 150 µg/kg stat, repeat every 6–12 months.[32]

and **antibiotics** to treat secondary bacterial infection if present.

> Reactions due to dying parasites are common and may commence a few hours after treatment. Worse in Brugian filariasis.

FOLLOW UP

Neither DEC nor ivermectin are particularly effective in killing adult worms, although efficacy is probably greater in *B. malayi* than *W. bancrofti* infections. Therefore repeat therapy may be necessary. Monitor the clinical course and repeat blood smears for microfilariae.

DRUG AVAILABILITY IN AUSTRALIA

Diethylcarbamazine   *Hetrazan:* 50 mg tabs
Ivermectin   *Stromectol:* 6 mg tabs

Appendix 1

Classification and biology of parasites

Classification

The term 'parasite' usually applies to a weaker organism that obtains food and shelter from another organism. Medical parasitology deals with animal parasites that infect the human host and may cause a range of health problems.

The animal parasites of humans are broadly divided into two groups:

Protozoa unicellular or acellular animals (they have the organelles of eucaryotic cells and may have more than one nucleus)

Metazoa multicellular animals (helminths, arthropods).

Each parasite belongs to a phylum, class, order, family, genus and species. Further divisions of subclass, suborder, superfamily, subfamily and subspecies are sometimes used. The names of genera and species are printed in italics; the generic name begins with a capital and the specific name with a small letter; for example, *Taenia solium*.

Parasite hosts are divided into definitive, intermediate, incidental and reservoir hosts.

Definitive contains the adult or the sexual stage of the parasite (e.g. humans are the definitive host for schistosomes, and the mosquito is for plasmodia).

Intermediate contains part or all of the larval or asexual stage of the parasite (e.g. the snail is the intermediate host for schistosomes, and the human is for malaria).

Incidental not necessary for the parasite's survival, but incidental (or accidental) infection may occur (e.g. humans infected with *Gnathostoma*).

Reservoir other animals that harbour the same parasite (e.g. cattle and wild animals for *Trypanosoma brucei rhodesiense*) and act as a potential source of human infection.

Protozoa

Protozoa are unicellular, but are more complex and larger than bacteria. Some are parasites of animals and humans, but the majority

133

Table 1 Overview of the protozoal infections of humans and their relative importance in terms of pathogenicity and distribution

	Important pathogens	Less important pathogens	Commensals
Amoebae	*Entamoeba histolytica* *Naegleria fowleri*	*Acanthamoeba* spp. *Blastocystis hominis*	*Entamoeba coli* *Entamoeba hartmanni* *Endolimax nana* *Iodamoeba butschlii*
Flagellates			
Intestinal flagellates of GIT and GUT	*Giardia duodenalis*	*Dientamoeba fragilis* *Trichomonas vaginalis*	*Chilomastix mesnili* *Trichomonas* spp.
Visceral flagellates of blood and tissues	*Trypanosoma* spp. *Leishmania* spp.		
Ciliates		*Balantidium coli*	
Apicomplexa			
Sporozoa	*Plasmodium* spp. *Toxoplasma gondii*	*Babesia* spp. *Isospora* spp.	
Coccidia	*Cryptosporidium parvum* *Cyclospora cayetanensis*	*Sarcocystis* spp.	
Microspora		The common human pathogens are *Enterocytozoon bieneusi* and *Encephalitozoon intestinalis*.	

are free living (Table 1). Protozoa, in contrast to helminths, usually multiply in their hosts and so disease may be initiated from only a few organisms. In general, they have a highly developed reproductive capacity, which aids their survival. Reproduction in the parasitic protozoa may be sexual or asexual. If necessary, protozoa survive transmission to another host by transforming into strong-walled cysts or by passing through an insect vector.

Protozoa are usually found in:

- the blood (e.g. malaria)
- the gut (e.g. *Giardia*, amoebae, *Cryptosporidium*), or
- the tissues (e.g. toxoplasma, *Leishmania*).

Protozoa can be classified as follows:

- **Amoebae** are primitive and usually dwell in the large intestine. Movement is by pseudopodia. *Entamoeba histolytica* is the most important pathogen in this group.
- **Flagellates** move by filamentous processes.
- **Ciliates** move by short hairs or cilia.
- **Apicomplexa** have no typical organs of locomotion. They have alternating sexual and asexual cycles of multiplication. This group includes the subclasses Coccidia (e.g. *Toxoplasma gondii*) and Sporozoa (e.g. plasmodia).
- **Microspora** are primitive intracellular parasites with minute characteristic spores (1–4 μm) and an inoculation tube.
- Unknown classification. *Pneumocystis carinii*, although behaving in many regards like a protozoan, has been shown with mitochondrial gene and rRNA sequencing to be more characteristic of a fungus.

Metazoa

HELMINTHS (WORMS)

Helminths are large organisms, ranging from a few millimetres to 25 metres in length, with a complex structure. They usually have an outer protective coating and differentiated organs. The life cycle often involves two or more hosts. Helminths are generally unable to multiply in the human. They may live for months or years.

The infective stage gains entry by

- ingestion,
- penetration of skin by larvae, or
- injection by insect vectors.

Helminths can be divided into two phyla: Nemathelminthes and Platyhelminthes.

Nemathelminthes (nematodes or round worms)
Nematodes are the most common helminths to parasitise humans and it is estimated that 1.5 billion people are infected worldwide.

Nematodes are non-segmented worms that are usually long and cylindrical and vary in length from a few millimetres to over 1 metre. All nematodes that are parasitic in humans have separate sexes. Daily egg production ranges from very few (*Strongyloides stercoralis*) to more than 200 000 (*Ascaris lumbricoides*).

There is a great variation in life cycle stages and pathological sequelae found in humans. One way of classifying the nematodes is according to their need for an intermediate host (Table 2). They may also be classified by their final habitat in the human body.

- **Intestinal** The eggs and larvae of nematodes living in the intestinal tract are passed outside the body in the faeces or may be deposited on the perianal skin by the female worm. Eggs of some species are immediately infective (*Enterobius vermicularis*) whereas others may require an extended period of embryonation in the soil (e.g. *Ascaris lumbricoides*). In some cases the eggs hatch in the soil and then initiate infection by larval penetration of the human skin (e.g. *Strongyloides stercoralis*, hookworms).
- **Tissue** Apart from *Dracunculus medinensis* (guinea worm), the tissue nematodes are mostly parasites of other animals, and occasionally infect humans. In some cases the larvae cannot fully mature in the human host and wander aimlessly through internal organs or under the skin.
- **Filarial** The adult human filarial parasites may inhabit the lymphatic and circulatory systems, the subcutaneous or deep connective tissues, or serous cavities. The worms range from 2 to 50 cm in length. Several months after infection the adult females produce microfilariae (prelarvae), which may then be detected in blood or cutaneous tissues depending on the species. The periodicity of microfilariae in the peripheral blood varies with species (e.g. the microfilariae of *Wuchereria bancrofti* are usually found in the blood at night). Transmission occurs via the bites of blood-sucking arthropods that have become infected through ingesting microfilariae.

Platyhelminthes (flat worms)
Cestodes (tapeworms) Adult cestodes inhabit the GIT of vertebrates, and their larvae inhabit the tissues of vertebrates and

Table 2 Classification of Nemathelminthes

Mode of transmission	Important pathogens	Animal nematodes that may cause aberrant infections in humans
No intermediate host		
Via direct infection	*Enterobius vermicularis* (pinworm)	
Via soil maturation	*Ascaris lumbricoides* (round worm)	*Ancylostoma braziliense*
	hookworms (*Necator, Ancylostoma*)	*Toxocara canis*
	Strongyloides stercoralis (can also autoinfect)	
	Trichuris trichiura (whipworm)	
Intermediate host required		
Via meat		*Trichinella spiralis*
Via fish		*Anisakis* spp.
Via crustacea	*Dracunculus medinensis* (guinea worm, can also infect animals)	
Via molluscs		*Angiostrongylus cantonensis*
Via insect bites (filarial nematodes)	*Brugia malayi, Wuchereria bancrofti*	*Dirofilaria immitis*
	Onchocerca volvulus	

Table 3 Platyhelminthes that infect humans

Class	Important pathogens	Less important pathogens
Cestodes (tapeworms)	*Echinococcus granulosus*	*Diphyllobothrium latum*
	Taenia saginata, T. solium	*Hymenolepis nana*
Trematodes		
Blood flukes	*Schistosoma mansoni,*	*S. intercalatum*
	S. japonicum,	*S. mekongi*
	S. haematobium	
Intestinal flukes		*Fasciolopsis buski*
Lung flukes	*Paragonimus westermani*	
Liver flukes	*Fasciola hepatica*	
	Opisthorchis sinensis	other *Opisthorchis* spp.

invertebrates. With the exception of *Hymenolepis nana*, the common tapeworms of humans require one or more intermediate hosts in which the larval worm develops after the host's ingestion of the egg (Table 3). Adult worms consist of a head (scolex) and flat, segmented bodies, and they vary in length between 3 mm and 10 m. The egg-containing segments (proglottids) detach and are excreted. Most cestodes are hermaphrodites. The life span for some species is said to be as long as 20–25 years.

Trematodes (flukes) The trematode species that are parasitic in humans are flat, elongated and leaf shaped, varying in size from 1 mm to several centimetres. Nutrients are absorbed through the outer surface or integument. Adult flukes are usually hermaphrodites, the main exceptions being the schistosomes. Sexual reproduction in the adult is followed by asexual multiplication of the larval stages in snails.

Flukes may be classified according to their final habitat in the human body; that is, into blood, intestinal, hepatic and pulmonary flukes (Table 3).

ARTHROPODS

This group of metazoa includes **ectoparasites**, which live on or in the skin. Diseases may be caused by ectoparasites (e.g. scabies, lice infestations, myiasis) or transmitted by ectoparasites (e.g. malaria, filariasis, leishmaniasis, trypanosomiasis). In the latter case the ectoparasite is referred to as a vector.

Appendix 2

Geographical distribution of parasites

Each parasite is listed below against the geographical areas where it occurs most commonly or where it has mostly been reported. Parasites may occasionally be reported from other areas. For a more detailed discussion on epidemiology see the individual parasite entry.

Africa *Diphyllobothrium, Dracunculus, Fasciola gigantica, Leishmania, Loa loa, Mansonella,* myiasis, *Onchocerca, Paragonimus westermani, Plasmodium* spp., *Schistosoma haematobium, S. intercalatum* and *S. mansoni, Spirometra, Strongyloides, Taenia, Trichostrongylus, Trypanosoma brucei, Wuchereria*

Central and South America *Angiostrongylus costaricensis, Anisakis, Balantidium, Diphyllobothrium, Leishmania, Mansonella,* myiasis, *Onchocerca, Paragonimus mexicanus, Plasmodium falciparum* and *P. vivax, Schistosoma mansoni, Spirometra, Taenia, Trypanosoma cruzi, Wuchereria*

Europe *Anisakis, Diphyllobothrium* (in Baltic countries), *Leishmania* and *Taenia* (in South), *Opisthorchis* (in East)

Indian subcontinent *Brugia, Fasciolopsis, Leishmania, Paragonimus westermani, Plasmodium falciparum* and *P. vivax, Strongyloides, Taenia, Wuchereria*

Japan *Anisakis, Capillaria, Diphyllobothrium, Gnathostoma, Opisthorchis, Spirometra, Trichostrongylus*

Middle East *Balantidium, Leishmania, Plasmodium falciparum* and *P. vivax, Schistosoma haematobium* and *S. mansoni, Wuchereria*

North America *Babesia*

Pacific Islands *Angiostrongylus cantonensis, Balantidium* (especially PNG), *Brugia, Plasmodium falciparum* and *P. vivax, Wuchereria*

South East Asia *Angiostrongylus cantonensis, Brugia, Capillaria philippinensis, Fasciola gigantica, Fasciolopsis, Gnathostoma, Opisthorchis, Paragonimus westermani, Plasmodium falciparum* and *P. vivax, Schistosoma japonicum* and *S. mekongi, Spirometra, Strongyloides, Taenia, Trichostrongylus, Wuchereria*

Worldwide *Acanthamoeba, Ascaris, Blastocystis, Cryptosporidium, Cyclospora, Dientamoeba, Echinococcus, Entamoeba, Enterobius, Fasciola hepatica, Giardia,* hookworms, *Hymenolepis,* microsporidia, *Naegleria, Pediculus, Phthirus, Pneumocystis, Sarcoptes, Toxocara, Toxoplasma, Trichinella, Trichomonas, Trichuris*

Appendix 3

Clinical presentations in parasitic infections

Parasites to be considered in diagnosis are listed below against the clinical presentation or systems/organs involved. For clinical details see the individual parasite entry.

Central nervous system *Acanthamoeba, Angiostrongylus,* cysticercosis, *Echinococcus, Entamoeba histolytica, Gnathostoma, Loa loa, Naegleria, Paragonimus, Plasmodium falciparum, Schistosoma japonicum, Schistosoma mansoni, Spirometra, Toxoplasma, Trichinella, Trypanosoma brucei*

Eye *Acanthamoeba, Angiostrongylus,* cysticercosis, *Dirofilaria, Gnathostoma, Leishmania, Loa loa,* microsporidia, myiasis, *Onchocerca, Spirometra, Toxocara, Toxoplasma, Trichinella, Trypanosoma cruzi*

Fever (PUO) *Brugia, Babesia, Entamoeba histolytica* (abscess), *Leishmania, Mansonella, Plasmodium* spp., *Toxocara, Toxoplasma, Trichinella, Schistosoma, Trypanosoma, Wuchereria*

Gastrointestinal tract *Angiostrongylus costaricensis, Anisakis, Ascaris, Balantidium, Capillaria, Cryptosporidium, Cyclospora, Dientamoeba, Diphyllobothrium, Entamoeba, Enterobius, Fasciolopsis, Giardia, Gnathostoma,* hookworms, *Hymenolepis, Isospora,* microsporidia, myiasis, *Paragonimus, Schistosoma, Strongyloides, Taenia, Trichinella, Trichostrongylus, Trichuris*

Genito-urinary tract (including STD) *Brugia, Phthirus, Schistosoma haematobium, Trichomonas, Wuchereria*

History of passing a worm *Ascaris, Taenia*

Liver and biliary tract *Babesia, Capillaria, Echinococcus, Entamoeba histolytica, Fasciola, Leishmania, Opisthorchis, Plasmodium* spp., *Schistosoma, Trypanosoma cruzi*

Lymphadenopathy *Brugia, Leishmania, Toxoplasma, Trypanosoma, Wuchereria*

Muscle cysticercosis, *Echinococcus,* microsporidia, *Trichinella*

Respiratory system *Ascaris, Capillaria, Dirofilaria, Echinococcus, Entamoeba histolytica,* hookworms, *Paragonimus, Pneumocystis, Strongyloides, Wuchereria*

Skin and mucous membrane *Acanthamoeba, Ancylostoma,* cysticercosis, *Dracunculus, Gnathostoma,* hookworms, *Leishmania, Loa loa, Mansonella,* myiasis, *Onchocerca, Pediculus, Phthirus, Sarcoptes, Schistosoma, Spirometra, Strongyloides, Toxocara, Trichinella, Trypanosoma*

Appendix 4

Antiparasitic drugs and parasites for which they are used

In general, protozoal infections require species-specific treatment. Metronidazole or tinidazole are effective for treating giardiasis, amoebiasis and trichomoniasis.

METAZOA

Although species-specific prescription of medication is still required, general rules of treatment apply according to phyla and class.

HELMINTHS

Nematodes
- Intestinal: albendazole, mebendazole
- Tissue: albendazole, mebendazole, thiabendazole (but may not be very responsive)
- Filarial: diethylcarbamazine, ivermectin

Cestodes
- Albendazole, niclosamide, praziquantel

Trematodes
- Praziquantel, triclabendazole

ECTOPARASITES
- Ivermectin, 1% or 5% permethrin

For details of usage, dosage and availability in Australia, see the individual parasite entry.

The following table is a complete list of anti-parasitic drugs used for various parasites.

Drug (generic name)	Trade name	Target parasite
Albendazole	Zentel, Eskazole	*Ancylostoma, Ascaris, Capillaria, Echinococcus, Enterobius, Gnathostoma, hookworms, microsporidia★, Strongyloides, Toxocara, Trichinella, Trichostrongylus, Trichuris*
Amphotericin B	Fungizone	*Acanthamoeba★, Leishmania, Naegleria★*
Amphotericin B (liposomal)	AmBisome	*Leishmania*
Artemether, Artesunate		*Plasmodium falciparum*
Atovaquone	Mepron	*Pneumocystis, Toxoplasma*
Atovaquone + proguanil	Malarone	*Plasmodium falciparum*
Azithromycin	Zithromax	*Cryptosporidium★, Toxoplasma*
Benzidazole	Rochagan	*Trypanosoma cruzi★*
Benzyl benzoate	Ascabiol	*Pediculus corporis, Sarcoptes*
Bithionol	Bitin	*Fasciola*
Chlorhexidine aqueous irrigations		*Acanthamoeba*
Chloroquine	Chlorquin	*Plasmodium vivax, P. malariae, P. ovale*
Clindamycin	Dalacin C	*Babesia, Toxoplasma*
Clotrimazole	Canesten	*Trichomonas*
Crotamiton	Eurax	*Sarcoptes*
Dapsone	Dapsone 100	*Pneumocystis*
Diethylcarbamazine (DEC)	Hetrazan	*Brugia, Loa loa, Mansonella streptocerca, Toxocara, Wuchereria*

Drug	Brand	Parasite
Diiodohydroxyquin or iodoquinol	Yodoxin	*Dientamoeba*
Diloxanide furoate	Furamide, Furosemide	*Entamoeba histolytica*
Doxycycline	Doryx, Vibramycin	*Dientamoeba, Plasmodium falciparum*
Eflornithine or DFMO	Ornidyl	*Trypanosoma brucei*
Fumagillin B		microsporidia
Halofantrine	Halfan	*Plasmodium falciparum* (not recommended)
Iodoquinol or diiodohydroxyquin	Yodoxin	*Dientamoeba*
Itraconazole	Sporonox	*Acanthamoeba, Leishmania*
Ivermectin	Stromectol	*Ancylostoma, Brugia, Loa loa, Mansonella ozzardi, Onchocerca, Sarcoptes, Strongyloides, Wuchereria*
Ketoconazole	Nizoral	*Leishmania*
Maldison	Cleensheen, Lice Rid	*Pediculus capitis*
Mebendazole	Vermox, Sqworm, Banworm	*Angiostrongylus*★, *Anisakis*★ *Ascaris, Capillaria, Enterobius, Gnathostoma, hookworms, Mansonella perstans, Trichinella, Trichuris*
Mefloquine	Lariam	*Plasmodium falciparum, P. vivax*
Meglumine antimoniate	Glucantim	*Leishmania*
Melarsoprol	Arsobal, Mel B	*Trypanosoma brucei*
Metronidazole	Flagyl, Metrogyl	*Balantidium, Blastocystis*★, *Dientamoeba fragilis, Dracunculus, Entamoeba histolytica, Giardia, Trichomonas*
Miconazole	Daktarin	*Acanthamoeba, Naegleria*

★ Unproven efficacy or unsatisfactory outcome (see the parasite entry for details).

Drug (generic name)	Trade name	Target parasite
Neomycin + polymyxin B + gramicidin	Neosporin	Acanthamoeba
Niclosamide	Yomesan	Diphyllobothrium, Fasciolopsis, Hymenolepis nana, Taenia
Nifurtimox	Lampit	Trypanosoma cruzi*
Octreotide	Sandostatin	microsporidia
Oxamniquin	Vansil	Schistosoma mansoni
Paromomycin	Humatin	Cryptosporidium*, Dientamoeba, Entamoeba histolytica, Giardia
Pentamidine isethionate		Leishmania, Pneumocystis, Trypanosoma brucei
Permethrin 1%	Pyrifoam, Nix Quellada Creme Quellada Lotion,	Pediculus capitis, Phthirus pubis
Permethrin 5%		Sarcoptes Lyclear
Piperazine citrate		Ascaris
Polyhexamethylene biguanide (PHMB) 0.02%		Acanthamoeba
Praziquantel	Biltricide	Diphyllobothrium, Echinococcus, Fasciolopsis, Hymenolepis nana, Opisthorchis, Paragonimus, Schistosoma, Taenia
Primaquine phosphate		Plasmodium vivax, P. falciparum gametocytes
Propamidine isethionate	Brolene eye drops	Acanthamoeba, microsporidia

Pyrantel embonate	*Anthel, Early Bird, Combantrin*	*Ascaris*, hookworms, *Trichostrongylus*
Pyrethrin + piperonyl butoxide	*Banlice Mousse, Lyban Foam*	*Pediculus, Phthirus*
Pyrimethamine	*Daraprim*	*Toxoplasma*
Pyrimethamine–sulfadoxine	*Fansidar*	*Plasmodium falciparum*
Quinine sulfate	*Quinate*	*Plasmodium falciparum, P. vivax*
Quinine dihydrochloride		*Plasmodium falciparum*
Spiramycin	*Rovamycin*	*Toxoplasma*
Stibogluconate sodium	*Pentostam*	*Leishmania*
Sulfadiazine		*Acanthamoeba, Toxoplasma*
Suramin		*Trypanosoma brucei*
Tetracycline	*Tetrex*	*Balantidium*
Thiabendazole	*Mintezol*	*Acanthamoeba, Angiostrongylus* *, Dracunculus, Strongyloides*
Tinidazole	*Fasigyn, Simplotan*	*Entamoeba histolytica, Giardia, Trichomonas*
Triclabendazole	*Fasinex*	*Fasciola*
Trimethoprim	*Triprim*	*Pneumocystis*
Trimethoprim–sulfamethoxazole	*Bactrim, Co-trimoxazole* solution, *Septrin*	*Cyclospora, Isospora, Pneumocystis*

* Unproven efficacy or unsatisfactory outcome (see the parasite entry for details).

Appendix 5

Access to unapproved drugs via the Special Access Scheme

Special Access Scheme (SAS) drugs are not registered in Australia, and the Commonwealth department (Department of Health Services and Health) does not give assurances of their quality, safety or efficacy.

Doctors wishing to apply for a drug to be placed on the SAS list should put an application in writing to the Drug Safety and Evaluation Branch (see below), giving details of the proposed use, an assurance that conventional therapy has failed or is not available, and any relevant information available about the drug. Such applications are considered at meetings of the senior medical officers of the Branch. The Branch evaluates applications to market new drugs for quality, safety and efficacy. It is not able to provide any information about drugs not registered in Australia.

Guidelines, application forms and lists of drugs available on SAS may be obtained from your hospital pharmacy or from the Information Officer, Therapeutic Goods Administration.

Drug Safety and Evaluation Branch
Therapeutic Goods Administration
PO Box 100
Woden ACT 2606

Phone: (02) 6232 8444 or 1800 020 653; Fax: (02) 6232 8241
E-mail: tga-information-officer@health.gov.au
Website: www.health.gov.au/tga/contacts.htm

Appendix 6

Useful addresses and contacts

Australian Capital Territory
  Special Access Scheme Approval
  Therapeutic Goods Administration
  PO Box 100
  Woden
  ACT 2606
  Australia
  Tel: 61 2 6232 8444; Fax: 61 2 6232 8241

New South Wales
  Centre for Infectious Diseases and Microbiology (CIDM)
  Westmead Hospital
  Westmead
  NSW 2145
  Australia
  Tel: 61 2 9845 7191; Fax: 61 2 9891 5317

  Dr John Walker
  Department of Parasitology
  Centre for Infectious Diseases and Microbiology
  Westmead Hospital
  Westmead
  NSW 2145
  Australia
  Tel: 61 2 9845 7663; Fax: 61 2 9891 5317
  E-mail: johnw@cidm.wh.usyd.edu.au

Queensland
  Associate Professor Paul Prociv
  Department of Parasitology
  The University of Queensland, Brisbane
  Qld 4072
  Australia
  Tel: 61 7 3365 3306; Fax: 61 7 3365 1588
  E-mail: p.prociv@mailbox.uq.oz.au

Associate Professor Rick Speare
School of Public Health and Tropical Medicine
James Cook University
Townsville
Qld 4811
Australia
Tel: 61 7 4722 5777 (direct) or 61 747 225 700 (department
  secretary); Fax: 61 7 4722 5788
E-mail: richard.speare@jcu.edu.au

Victoria
Dr Beverley-Ann Biggs
Department of Medicine
The University of Melbourne
The Royal Melbourne Hospital
Parkville
Vic. 3050
Australia
Tel: 61 3 9344 5478 or 61 3 9344 5479; Fax: 61 3 9347 1896
E-mail: biggs@wehi.edu.au

Dr Harsha Sheorey
Department of Microbiology
St Vincent's Hospital
Fitzroy
Vic. 3065
Australia
Tel: 61 3 9288 4066; Fax 61 3 9288 4068
E-mail: sheoreyh@australiamail.com

Microbiological Diagnostic Unit
Department of Microbiology and Immunology
The University of Melbourne
Parkville
Vic. 3052
Australia
Tel: 61 3 9344 5701; Fax: 61 3 9344 7833

Paraclinical Sciences
The University of Melbourne, Werribee Campus
50 Princes Highway
Werribee
Vic. 3030
Australia
Tel: 61 3 741 3500; Fax: 61 3 741 0401

Victorian Infectious Diseases Reference Laboratory (VIDRL)
Locked Bag 815
Carlton South
Vic. 3053
Australia
Tel: 61 3 9342 2600; Fax 61 3 9342 2665

Victorian Infectious Diseases Service
The Royal Melbourne Hospital
Parkville
Vic. 3050
Australia
Tel: 61 3 9342 7212; Fax: 61 3 9342 7277

INTERNATIONAL

Center for Disease Control (CDC)
Division of Parasitic Diseases
Chamblee 102
Atlanta GA
USA
Tel: 1 1 770 488 7750; Fax: 1 1 770 488 7794

USEFUL INTERNET SITES

For parasitic diseases

http://www.dpd.cdc.gov/DPDx

http://www.dpd.cdc.gov/DPDx/HTML/Para_Health.htm

http://www.who.int/home/map_ht.html

For tropical diseases

http://pathcuric1.swmed.edu/microbiology/labref/Parasites/
ParaimageTofC.html

http://www.cdfound.to.it/html/atlas.htm#atlas

ProMED mail Post
http://www.promedmail.org:8080/promed/promed.folder.home

Glossary

µg micrograms

µm micrometres (microns)

accidental host unnatural host that gets infected accidentally; the life cycle of the parasite is interrupted

adult worms mature forms of helminths

AIDS acquired immune deficiency syndrome

amastigote small oval intracellular stage of *Leishmania* spp., also called LD bodies

amoeba unicellular organism that moves by pseudopodia

BAL bronchoalveolar lavage

caps capsules

CDC Center for Disease Control (*see* Appendix 6)

cercariae free-living, tailed, larval stage of trematodes

cestodes tapeworms; helminths with a flat tape-like body

chagoma small granuloma seen in Chagas' disease

CIDM Centre for Infectious Diseases and Microbiology

CLB cyanobacterium-like bodies, term previously used for *Cyclospora* spp.

CLM cutaneous larva migrans

CNS central nervous system

creeping eruptions penetration and migration of larvae of some nematodes (e.g. *Strongyloides*, hookworms) through the sub-cutaneous tissue, resulting in intense pruritis

CSF cerebrospinal fluid

CT computed tomography

CXR chest X-ray

cysticercus bladder-shaped larval form of tapeworms

cysts infective stage of protozoa, which have a thick outer wall to overcome harsh environmental conditions

DEC diethylcarbamazine

definitive host host in which the sexual cycle of the parasite occurs or in which adult/mature forms are seen

diurnal pertaining to daytime

DS double strength

ECG electrocardiograph

eggs/ova laid by adult female (nematodes) or hermaphroditic worms (cestodes and trematodes); diagnostic form in a number of parasites

EIA enzyme immuno-assay; same as ELISA

elephantiasis hypertrophy of tissues due to chronic obstruction of the lymphatic ducts in filariasis

endoparasite parasite living within the body of a host

ENT ear, nose and throat

Entero-Test special test for collecting upper GIT material. It consists of a capsule (containing absorbent material inside) at the end of a thread, which is swallowed by the patient until the capsule reaches the duodenum or jejunum, where it is left for a while to absorb the contents, and then pulled out by the thread in the mouth.

ESR erythrocyte sedimentation rate

exoparasite parasite that lives on the surface of a host (e.g. lice, mites)

faecal concentration technique used to increase the yield of parasites in a faecal sample

FBC full blood count

filariform larvae infective stage in the development of *Strongyloides* and hookworms

g grams

gametocyte sexual stage in the malarial parasite; both male and female gametocytes are present

GIT gastrointestinal tract

GUT genito-urinary tract

helminths nematodes, cestodes or trematodes

HIV human immunodeficiency virus

hookworms nematodes possessing hook-like structures in the mouth to hold on to host tissue

hydatid sand part of the hydatid fluid found in the cyst of *Echinococcus granulosus*, consisting of scolices, hooks and daughter cysts

ICT immunochromatographic test

IEP immunoelectrophoresis

IFA indirect fluorescent antibody

IHA indirect haemagglutination test

im intramuscular

inj injection

intermediate host host in which the larval or development stage is seen or in which the asexual cycle of the parasite occurs

iv intravenous

kala-azar visceral leishmaniasis (*kala* = black, *azar* = fever)

Knott concentration concentration technique for blood using dilute formalin

larva migrans (cutaneous, visceral, ocular) eruptions or involvement of tissue along the path of migrating larvae, usually of animal hookworms or roundworms

larvae/larval form developmental stage of helminths, which hatch out of eggs and become adults; can be infective and/or invasive

LD bodies Leishman-Donovan bodies, amastigote forms of *Leishmania* spp.

LIT Liver infusion tryptose medium (Yaeger's medium)

LFT liver function tests

max. maximum

Mazzoti reaction diagnostic test to enhance the rash of onchocerciasis by giving a single oral dose of DEC

merozoites stage in the cycle of the malarial parasite in humans

mg milligrams

microfilariae larval form of filarial worms found in the blood or tissue of the patient

miracidium free-living ciliated larval form of trematodes, infective for intermediate host (snails)

mL millilitres

MRI magnetic resonance imaging

myiasis infestation by larva or maggots of certain insects

nematodes helminths with a cylindrical body

New World Western hemisphere; mainly the Americas

NNN Novy, MacNeal and Nicolle's medium

nocturnal pertaining to night-time

NPA nasopharyngeal aspirate

OD optical density (measurement used in EIA)

Old World Eastern hemisphere; Europe, Africa, Asia

OLM ocular larva migrans

operculated eggs eggs with a lid-like structure at one end (e.g. some trematodes)

optimal host the natural or usual host

paratenic host transport host in which the parasite survives without undergoing any further development

PCR polymerase chain reaction

po per os (i.e. orally)

proglottids segments of tapeworms containing male and female reproductive organs; may be immature, mature or gravid (containing eggs)

promastigote developmental stage of trypanosomes

protozoa unicellular organisms that usually divide asexually by binary fission (except *Plasmodium* spp.)

PUO pyrexia of unknown origin

RBC red blood cells

reservoir host other animal that harbours the same parasite and acts as a potential source of human infection

rhabditiform larvae non-infective stage in the development of *Strongyloides* and hookworms

RLQ right lower quadrant

RUQ right upper quadrant

SAS Special Access Scheme (*see* Appendix 5)

sc subcutaneous

scolex head of the tapeworm, may have hooklets or suckers

Scotch tape/sticky tape prep. preparation for microscopic examination of eggs of *Enterobius vermicularis* by applying sticky tape on the anus of a child suffering from anal pruritis

sparganum larval form of *Spirometra* or *Diphyllobothrium* tapeworms

sporozoites infective stage of the malaria parasite, inoculated by the bite of an *Anopheles* mosquito

STD sexually transmitted disease

T+T smears thick and thin smears of peripheral blood (e.g. for malaria)

tabs tablets

trematodes flukes; helminths with a flat, usually leaf-shaped, body

trophozoites the feeding motile and/or invasive stage of protozoa; also the early to mid stage in the erythrocytic cycle of malaria

trypomastigote developmental stage of trypanosomes

U&E urea and electrolytes

VIDRL Victorian Infectious Diseases Reference Laboratory (*see* Appendix 6)

VLM visceral larva migrans

WCC white cell count

wet prep. wet preparation of a faecal specimen for microscopy using saline

WHO World Health Organization

xenodiagnosis concentration technique where laboratory-raised insects are fed with the blood of a suspected patient (e.g. in Chagas' disease) and later the faeces of the insect are examined for parasites

zoonosis a disease of animals that is transmissible to humans

References

1 Mandell G L, Bennett J E, Dolin R eds. *Mandell, Douglas and Bennett's Principles and Practice of Infectious Disease*, 4th edn, New York: Churchill Livingstone, 1995.

2 Garcia L S, Bruckner D A eds. *Diagnostic Medical Parasitology*, 3rd edn, Washington: ASM Press, 1997.

3 Cook G C ed. *Manson's Tropical Diseases*, 20th edn, London: Saunders, 1996.

4 Therapeutic Guidelines Limited. *Therapeutic Guidelines: Antibiotic*, 10th edn, Melbourne: TGL, 1998–99.

5 Slater C A, Sickel J Z, Visvesvara G S, Pabico R C, Gaspari A A. Successful treatment of disseminated Acanthamoeba infection in an immunocompromised patient. *New England Journal of Medicine* 1994, **331:** 85–7.

6 Murakawa G J, McCalmont T, Altman J, Telang G H, Hoffman M D, Kantor G R et al. Disseminated acanthamebiasis in patients with AIDS. *Archives of Dermatology* 1995, **131:** 1291–6.

7 Reed R P, Cooke-Yarborough C M, Jaquiery A L, Grimwood K, Kemp A S, Su J C et al. Fatal granulomatous amoebic encephalitis caused by *Balmuthia mandrillaris*. *Medical Journal of Australia* 1997, **167:** 82–4.

8 Department of Ophthalmology, The University of Melbourne (Royal Victorian Eye and Ear Hospital). Acanthamoeba keratitis protocol 1997, Feb.

9 Ishibashi Y, Matsumoto Y, Kabata T, Watanabe R, Hommura S, Yasuraoka K et al. Oral itraconazole and topical miconazole with debridement for *Acanthamoeba* keratitis. *American Journal of Ophthalmology* 1990, **109:** 121–6.

10 Croese L, Loukas A, Opdebeeck J, Prociv P. Occult enteric infection by *Ancylostoma caninum*: a previously unrecognized zoonosis. *Gastroenterology* 1994, **106:** 3–12.

11 Prociv P, Croese J. Human eosinophilic enteritis caused by dog hookworm *Ancylostoma caninum*. *Lancet* 1990, **335:** 1299–1302.

12 Jelinek T, Maiwald H, Nothdurft H D, Loscher T. Cutaneous larva migrans in travellers: synopsis of histories, symptoms, and treatment of 98 patients. *Clinical Infectious Diseases* 1994, **19:** 1062–6.

13 Simpson T W. More on *Angiostrongylus cantonensis* infection. *New England Journal of Medicine* 1995, **333:** 882.

14 Collins G H, Rothwell T L W, Malik R, Church D B, Dowden M K. Angiostrongylosis in dogs in Sydney. *Australian Veterinary Journal* 1992, **69:** 170–1.

15 Paine M, Davis S, Brown G. Severe forms of infection with *Angiostrongylus cantonensis* acquired in Australia and Fiji. *Australian and New Zealand Journal of Medicine* 1994, **24:** 415–16.

16 Zaman V. Other gut nematodes. In Weatherall D J, Ledingham J G G, Warrell D A eds. *Oxford Textbook of Medicine*, 3rd edn, vol. 1. Oxford: Oxford University Press, 1996, 938–9.

17 Gilbert D N, Moellering M D, Sande M A eds. *The Sanford Guide to Antimicrobial Therapy*, 28th edn, Vienna (USA): Antimicrobial Therapy, Inc., 1998.

18 Salman A B. Management of intestinal obstruction caused by ascariasis. *Journal of Paediatric Surgery* 1997, **32**: 585–7.

19 Radford A J. Balantidiasis in Papua New Guinea. *Medical Journal of Australia* 1973, **1**: 238–41.

20 Zierdt C H. *Blastocystis hominis:* past and future. *Clinical Microbiology Reviews* 1991, **4**: 61–79.

21 Shlim D R, Hoge C W, Rajah R, Rabold J G, Echeverria P. Is *Blastocystis hominis* a cause of diarrhea in travelers? A prospective controlled study in Nepal. *Clinical Infectious Diseases* 1995, **21**: 97–101.

22 Stenzel D J, Boreham P F L. *Blastocystis hominis* revisited. *Clinical Microbiology Reviews* 1996, **9**: 563–84.

23 Walker J C, Bahr G, Ehl A S. Gastrointestinal parasites in Sydney. *Medical Journal of Australia* 1985, **143**: 480.

24 Cross J H. Intestinal capillariasis [review]. *Clinical Microbiology Reviews* 1992, **5**: 120–9.

25 DuPont H L, Chappell C L, Sterling C R, Okhuysen P C, Rose J B, Jakubowski W et al. The infectivity of *Cryptosporidium parvum* in healthy volunteers. *New England Journal of Medicine* 1995, **332**: 855–9.

26 Lemmon J M, McAnulty J M, Bawden-Smith J. Outbreak of cryptosporidiosis linked to an indoor swimming pool. *Medical Journal of Australia* 1996, **165**: 613–16.

27 Cryptosporidiosis outbreak. *Communicable Diseases Intelligence* 1998, **22**: 22.

28 Cryptosporidiosis: Australia (Victoria). ProMED-mail post, 2 April 1998.

29 MacKenzie W R, Hoxie N J, Proctor M E, Gradus M S, Blair K A, Peterson D E et al. A massive outbreak in Milwaukee of cryptosporidium infection transmitted through the public water supply. *New England Journal of Medicine* 1994, **331**: 161–7.

30 Sarabia-Arce S, Salazar-Lindo E, Gilman R H, Naranjo J, Miranda E. Case control study of *Cryptosporidium parvum* infection in Peruvian children hospitalized for diarrhea: possible association with malnutrition and nosocomial infection. *Pediatric Infectious Disease Journal* 1990, **9**: 627–31.

31 Foodborne outbreak of diarrheal illness associated with *Cryptosporidium parvum. Morbidity and Mortality Weekly Report* 1996, **45**: 783–4.

32 Moellering R C, Maguire J H, Keystone J S eds. *Infectious Disease Clinics of North America: Parasitic Diseases*, vol. 7. Philadelphia: W B Saunders, 1993.

33 Liu L X, Weller P F. Antiparasitic drugs [review]. *New England Journal of Medicine* 1996, **334**: 1178–84.

34 Smith N H, Cron S, Valdez L M, Chappell C L, White A C Jr. Combination drug therapy for cryptosporidiosis in AIDS. *Journal of Infectious Diseases* 1998, **178**: 900–3.

35 Outbreaks of *Cyclospora cayetanensis* infection: United States and Canada, 1996. *Morbidity and Mortality Weekly Report* 1996, **45**: 611–12.

36 Pape J W, Verdier R I, Boncy M, Boncy J, Johnson W D Jr. Cyclospora infection in adults infected with HIV: Clinical manifestations, treatment and prophylaxis. *Annals of Internal Medicine* 1994, **121**: 654–7.

37 Sawangjaroen N, Luke R, Provic P. Diagnosis by faecal culture of *Dientamoeba fragilis* infections in Australian patients with diarrhoea. *Transactions of the Royal Society of Tropical Medicine and Hygiene* 1993, **87**: 163–5.

38 Boreham R E, Cooney P T, Stewart P A. Dirofilariasis with conjunctival inflammation [letter]. *Medical Journal of Australia* 1997, **167**: 51.

39 Hopkins D R, Azam M, Ruiz-Tiben E, Kappus K D. Eradication of dracunculiasis from Pakistan. *Lancet* 1995, **346**: 621–4.

40 Imported dracunculiasis: United States, 1995 and 1997. *Morbidity and Mortality Weekly Report* 1998, **47**: 209–11.

41 Walker J. Hydatid disease [seminar]. *Inoculum* (Newsletter of CIDM, IPCMR, Westmead Hospital, Sydney) March 1995, 1–3.

42 Thompson R C A, Lymbery A J, Hobbs R P, Elliot A D. Hydatid disease in urban areas of Western Australia: an unusual cycle involving western grey kangaroos (*Macropus fuliginosus*), feral pigs and domestic dogs. *Australian Veterinary Journal* 1988, **65**: 188–90.

43 Jenkins D J, Power K. Human hydatidosis in New South Wales and the Australian Capital Territory, 1987–1992. *Medical Journal of Australia* 1996, **164**: 18–21.

44 Lightowlers M W (Molecular Parasitology Laboratory, University of Melbourne, Werribee Campus). Laboratory diagnosis of hydatid disease [seminar at Westmead Hospital, Sydney] March 1995.

45 Filice C, Brunetti E. Echo-guided diagnosis and treatment of hepatic hydatid cysts. *Clinical Infectious Diseases* 1997, **25**: 169–71.

46 Craig P S, Deshan L, MacPherson C N, Dazhong S, Reynolds D, Barnish G et al. A large focus of alveolar echinococcosis in central China. *Lancet* 1992, **340**: 826–31.

47 Law C L H, Walker J, Qassim M H. Factors associated with detection of *Entamoeba histolytica* in homosexual men. *International Journal of STD and AIDS* 1991, **2**: 346–50.

48 Torresi J, Richards M J, Taggart G J, Smallwood R A. *Fasciola hepatica* liver infection in a Victorian dairy farmer [letter]. *Medical Journal of Australia* 1996, **164**: 511.

49 Laird P P, Boray J C. Human fascioliasis successfully treated with triclabendazole. *Australian and New Zealand Journal of Medicine* 1992, **22**: 45–7.

50 Apt W, Aguilera X, Vega F, Miranda C, Zulantay I, Perez C et al. Treatment of human chronic fascioliasis with triclabendazole: drug efficiency and serologic response. *American Journal of Tropical Medicine and Hygiene* 1995, **52**: 532–5.

51 Butcher A R, Talbot G A, Norton R E, Kirk M D, Cribb T H, Forsyth J R L et al. Locally acquired *Brachylaima* spp. (*Digenea: Brachylaimidae*) intestinal fluke infection in two South Australian infants. *Medical Journal of Australia* 1996, **164**: 475–8.

52 Prociv P, Luke R A. The changing epidemiology of human hookworm infection in Australia [review]. *Medical Journal of Australia* 1995, **162**: 150–4.

53 Hopkins R M, Gracey M S, Hobbs R P, Spargo R M, Yates M, Thompson R C A. The prevalence of hookworm infection, iron deficiency and anaemia in an Aboriginal community in northwest Australia. *Medical Journal of Australia* 1997, **166**: 241–4.

54 Reynoldson J A, Behnke J M, Pallant L J, Macnish M G, Gilbert F, Giles S et al. Failure of pyrantel in treatment of human hookworm infections in the Kimberley region of northwest Australia. *Acta Tropica* 1997, **68**: 301–12.

55 Visvanathan K, Jones P D, Riordan S M, Thomas M C. Delayed reactivation of visceral leishmaniasis complicating HIV infection. *Australian and New Zealand Journal of Medicine* 1993, **23**: 407.

56 Lee M B, Gilbert H M. Current approaches to leishmaniasis. *Infections in Medicine* 1999, **16**: 34–45.

57 Gradoni L, Bryceson A, Desjeux P. Treatment of Mediterranean visceral leishmaniasis. *Bulletin of the World Health Organization* 1995, **73**: 191–7.

58 Mishra M, Biswas U K, Jha A M, Khan A B. Amphotericin versus sodium stibogluconate in first-line treatment in Indian kala-azar. *Lancet* 1994, **344**: 1599–1600.

59 Momeni A Z, Jalayer T, Emamjomeh M, Bashardost N, Ghassemi R L, Meghdadi M et al. Treatment of cutaneous leishmaniasis with itraconazole. *Archives of Dermatology* 1996, **132**: 784–6.

60 Navin T R, Arana B A, Arana F E, Berman J D, Chajon J F. Placebo controlled clinical trial of sodium stibogluconate (Pentostam) versus ketoconazole for treating cutaneous leishmaniasis in Guatemala. *Journal of Infectious Diseases* 1992, **165**: 528–34.

61 Melby P C, Kreutzer R D, McMahon-Pratt D, Gam A A, Neva F A. Cutaneous leishmaniasis: review of 59 cases seen at NIH. *Clinical Infectious Diseases* 1992, **15**: 924–37.

62 Ng S O C, Yates M. Cutaneous myiasis in a traveller returning from Africa. *Australian Journal of Dermatology* 1997, **38**: 38–9.

63 Lukin L. Human cutaneous myiasis in Brisbane: a prospective study. *Medical Journal of Australia* 1989, **150**: 237–40.

64 Bryan R T, Weber R, Schwartz D A. Microsporidiosis in patients who are not infected with human immunodeficiency virus [letter]. *Clinical Infectious Diseases* 1997, **24**: 534–5.

65 Field A S, Marriott D J, Milliken S T, Brew B J, Canning E U, Kench J G et al. Myositis associated with a newly described microsporidian, *Trachipleistophora hominis*, in a patient with AIDS. *Journal of Clinical Microbiology* 1996, **34**: 2803–11.

66 Ryan N J, Sutherland G, Coughlan K, Globan M, Doultree J, Marshall J et al. A new Trichrome-blue stain for detection of microsporidial species in urine, stool and nasopharyngeal specimen. *Journal of Clinical Microbiology* 1993, **31:** 3264–9.

67 Sobottka I, Albrecht H, Schafer H, Schottelius J, Visvesvara G S, Laufs R et al. Disseminated *Encephalitozoon (Septata) intestinalis* infection in a patient with AIDS: novel diagnostic approaches and autopsy-confirmed parasitological cure following treatment with albendazole. *Journal of Clinical Microbiology* 1995, **33:** 2948–52.

68 Didier E S. Microsporidiosis [state-of-the-art clinical article]. *Clinical Infectious Diseases* 1998, **27:** 1–8.

69 Knight R. Amoebiasis. In Weatherall D J, Ledingham J G G, Warrell D A, eds. *Oxford Textbook of Medicine*, 3rd edn, vol. 1. Oxford: Oxford University Press, 1996, 825–34.

70 Leichsenring M, Troger J, Nelle M, Buttner D W, Darge K, Doehring-Schwerdtfeger E. Ultrasonographical investigations of onchocerciasis in Liberia. *American Journal of Tropical Medicine and Hygiene* 1990, **43:** 380–5.

71 Speare R. Head Lice Information Sheet. Department of Public Health and Tropical Medicine, James Cook University, Townsville, Queensland, 1999 Feb. (Available from: http://www.jcu.edu.au/dept/PHTM/hlice/hlinfo1.htm)

72 Jenkin G A, Ritchie S A, Hanna J N, Brown G V. Airport malaria in Cairns. *Medical Journal of Australia* 1997, **166:** 307–8.

73 Tjitra E, Suprianto S, Dyer M, Currie B J, Anstey N M. Field evaluation of the ICT malaria P.f/P.v immunochromatographic test for detection of plasmodium falciparum and plasmodium vivax in patients with a presumptive clinical diagnosis of malaria in Eastern Indonesia. *Journal of Clinical Microbiology* 1999, **37:** 2412–17.

74 Rogerson S J, Biggs B A, Brown G V. Chemoprophylaxis and treatment of malaria [review]. *Australian Family Physician* 1994, **23:** 1696–709.

75 Yung A, Ruff T A. *Manual of Travel Medicine: a guide for practitioners at pre-travel clinics*. Victorian Infectious Diseases Service, Royal Melbourne Hospital Fairfield Travel Health Clinic, 1999.

76 Davis T M E, Breheny F X, Kendall P A, Daly F, Batty K T, Singh A et al. Severe falciparum malaria with hyperparasitaemia treated with intravenous artesunate. *Medical Journal of Australia* 1997, **166:** 416–18.

77 Lewin S R, Hoy J, Crowe S M, McDonald C F. The role of bronchoscopy in the diagnosis and treatment of pulmonary disease in HIV infected patients. *Australian and New Zealand Journal of Medicine* 1995, **25:** 133–9.

78 Fishman J A. Treatment of infection due to *Pneumocystis carinii*. *Antimicrobial Agents and Chemotherapy* 1998, **42:** 1309–14.

79 Speare R, McConnell A. *Sarcoptes scabei* resistant to permethrin. In *Proceedings of the 5th Annual Scientific Meeting of the Australasian College of Tropical Medicine*, 14–17 June 1996. Townsville: ACTM Publication, 28.

80 Meinking T L, Taplin D, Hermida J L, Pardo R, Kerdel F A. The treatment of scabies with ivermectin. *New England Journal of Medicine* 1995, **333:** 26–30.

81 Barkwell R, Shields S. Deaths associated with ivermectin treatment of scabies. *Lancet* 1997, **349:** 1144–5.

82 Hipgrave D B, Leydon J A, Walker J, Biggs B A. Schistosomiasis in Australian travellers to Africa. *Medical Journal of Australia* 1997, **166:** 294–7.

83 Torresi J, Sheorey H, Ryan N, Yung A. The usefulness of semen microscopy in the diagnosis of a difficult case of *Schistosoma haematobium* infection in a returned traveller. *Journal of Travel Medicine* 1997, **4:** 46–7.

84 Gui M, Idris M A, Shi Y E, Muhling A, Ruppel A. Reactivity of *Schistosoma japonicum* and *S. mansoni* antigen preparations in indirect haemagglutination (IHA) with sera of patients with homologous and heterologous schistosomiasis. *Annals of Tropical Medicine and Parasitology* 1991, **85:** 599–604.

85 Murray-Smith S Q, Scott B J, Barton D P, Weinstein P. A case of refractory schistosomiasis [letter]. *Medical Journal of Australia* 1996, **165:** 458.

86 Hipgrave D B. A case of refractory schistosomiasis. *Medical Journal of Australia* 1997, **166:** 567.

87 Davis T M E, Beaman M H, McCarthy J S. Schistosomiasis in Australian travellers to Africa [letter]. *Medical Journal of Australia* 1998, **168:** 47.

88 Biggs B A, Yung A, Ruff T, Hipgrave D B. Schistosomiasis in Australian travellers to Africa [reply to letter]. *Medical Journal of Australia* 1998, **168:** 47.

89 Manoury V, Guillemot F, Mathieu-Chandelier C, Dutoit E, Gower-Rousseau C, Cortot A et al. Bilharzioses à *Schistosoma mekongi* diagnostiquées par biopsie rectale et traitées par praziquantel: à propos de 5 cases. *Gastroenterologie Clinique Biologique* 1990, **14:** 1032–3.

90 Munckhof W J, Grayson M L, Susil B J, Pullar M J, Turnidge J. Cerebral sparganosis in an East Timorese refugee. *Medical Journal of Australia* 1994, **161:** 263–4.

91 Lindo J F, Conway D J, Atkins N S, Bianco A E, Robinson R D, Bundy D A. Prospective evaluation of enzyme-linked immunosorbent assay and immunoblot for the diagnosis of endemic *Strongyloides stercoralis* infection. *American Journal of Tropical Medicine and Hygiene* 1994, **51:** 175–9.

92 White A C Jr. Neurocysticercosis: a major cause of neurological disease worldwide [state-of-the-art clinical article]. *Clinical Infectious Diseases* 1997, **24:** 101–13.

93 Evans C, Garcia H H, Gilman R H, Friedland J S. Controversies in management of cysticercosis. *Emerging Infectious Diseases* 1997, **3:** 403–5.

94 Zaman V. Toxocariasis and visceral larva migrans. In Weatherall D J, Ledingham J G G, Warrell D A eds. *Oxford Textbook of Medicine*, 3rd edn, vol. 1. Oxford: Oxford University Press, 1996, 944–5.

95 Hohlfeld P, Daffos F, Costa J M, Thulliez P, Forestier F, Vidaud M. Prenatal diagnosis of congenital toxoplasmosis with a polymerase-chain-reaction test on amniotic fluid. *New England Journal of Medicine* 1994, **331:** 695–9.

96 Bowden F, Hoy J, Mijch A, Robinson J eds. *Fairfield Hospital (Melbourne): HIV Medicine Handbook*, 2nd edn, Melbourne: Melbourne University Press, 1995.

97 Outbreak of trichinellosis associated with eating cougar jerky: Idaho, 1995. *Morbidity and Mortality Weekly Report* 1996, **45:** 205–6.

98 Jongwutiwes S, Chantachum N, Kraivichian P, Siriyasatien P, Putaporntip C, Tamburrini A et al. First outbreak of human trichinellosis caused by *Trichinella pseudospiralis. Clinical Infectious Diseases* 1998, **26:** 111–15.

99 Capo V, Despommier D D. Clinical aspects of infection with *Trichinella* spp. *Clinical Microbiology Reviews* 1996, **9:** 47–54.

100 Petrin D, Delgaty K, Bhatt R, Garber G. Clinical and microbiological aspects of *Trichomonas vaginalis* [review]. *Clinical Microbiology Reviews* 1998, **11:** 300–17.

101 Mackey S L, Wagner K F. Dermatologic manifestations of parasitic diseases. *Infectious Disease Clinics of North America* 1994, **8:** 713–43.

102 de Andrade A L S, Zicker F, de Oliveira R M, Almeida Silva S, Luquetti A, Travassos L R et al. Randomised trial of efficacy of benzidazole in treatment of early *Trypanosoma cruzi* infection. *Lancet* 1996, **348:** 1407–13.

Index

Acanthamoeba 1, 2, 70, 134, 139, 140, 142, 143, 144, 145
African eyeworm 59
AIDS 1, 17, 21, 53, 67, 90, 93, 115, 116
albendazole 5, 12, 20, 34, 35, 36, 40, 41, 47, 49, 51, 68, 69, 105, 106, 111, 113, 119, 122, 123, 124, 141, 142
amastigote forms 56, 151
amoeba 37, 150
  amoebiasis 37, 141
  amoebic colitis 15, 37
  amoebic dysentery 123
  amoebic encephalitis 1
  amoebic granulomas 1
  amoebic liver abscess 38
  amoeboid trophozoites 70
  extra-intestinal amoebiasis 37, 38
  free living amoebae 1, 70
  intestinal amoebiasis 25, 37, 38
  leptomyxid amoebae 1
  primary amoebic meningo-encephalitis (PAM) 70
amphotericin B 2, 3, 57, 58, 142
Ancylostoma braziliense 4, 136
Ancylostoma caninum 4–5
Ancylostoma duodenale see hookworm
Angiostrongylus cantonensis 6, 136
Angiostrongylus costaricensis 7, 139, 140
animal hookworms 4
Anisakis species 9, 136, 139, 140, 143
Anopheles species 83
antimony compounds 57, 58
Arachnida 93
artesunate 85
Ascaris 8, 11, 136, 137, 139, 140, 142, 143, 144, 145
atovaquone 85, 91, 142
azithromycin 22, 116, 142

Babesia microti 13, 134, 139, 140, 142
Balantidium coli 15, 134, 139, 140, 143, 145
beef tapeworm 107
benzyl benzoate 80, 94, 142
blackfly 72
Blastocystis hominis 17, 134, 139, 143
blood fluke 95, 138
blue-green algae 23
body louse 79
botfly 61
Brachylaima species 44
Brugia malayi 130, 132, 136, 139, 140, 142, 143

calabar swellings 59, 64
canine tapeworm 33
Capillaria philippinensis 19, 139, 140, 142, 144
cestode 33, 52, 107
Chagas' disease 56, 127, 128
Chinese or Oriental liver fluke 74
chlorhexidine 3, 142
chloroquine 85, 87, 88, 89, 142
Chrysomyia bezziana 61
Chrysops species 59
Clonorchis sinensis 74
clotrimazole 121, 142
Cochliomyia hominivorax 61
Cordylobia anthropophaga 61
corticosteroids 3, 7, 12, 43, 49, 60, 73, 77, 91, 93, 111, 113, 116, 119
co-trimoxazole 23, 92
crab/pubic louse *see* louse
creeping eruption 4
Cryptosporidium parvum 21, 134, 139, 140, 142, 144
Culicoides species 63–5
cutaneous larva migrans (CLM) 4–5
cutaneous leishmaniasis 57

cyanobacterium-like bodies (CLB) 23
Cyclospora cayetanensis 23–4, 134, 139, 145
cysticercus 7, 102, 107–11

deer fly 59
Dermatobium hominis 61
DFMO *see* eflornithine
Dientamoeba fragilis 25, 134, 139, 140, 143–4
diethylcarbamazine (DEC) 60, 64–6, 72–3, 113, 131–2, 141–2
diiodohydroxyquin 25, 143
diloxanide furoate 38, 39, 143
Diphyllobothrium latum 27, 138–40, 144
Dirofilaria immitis 29, 59, 63–6, 136, 140
doxycycline 25, 85, 88, 143
Dracunculus medinensis 31, 136, 139, 140, 143, 145
dwarf tapeworm 52

East African trypanosomiasis 125
Echinococcus 33, 139, 140, 142, 144
   E. granulosus 33, 138
   E. multilocularis 35
   E. vogeli 35
eflornithine 126, 143
Encephalitozoon cuniculi 67, 68–9
Encephalitozoon hellem 67, 68–9
Encephalitozoon (Septata) intestinalis 67, 68–9, 134
Entamoeba 134, 139
   E. coli 38
   E. dispar 37
   E. histolytica 37, 134, 140, 143
Entero-Test 47, 53, 105
Enterobius vermicularis 25, 40, 136, 139–40, 142–3
Enterocytozoon bieneusi 67–8, 134
enzyme immuno-assay (EIA) 7, 22, 34, 38, 43, 47, 59, 63–6, 73, 97, 99, 105, 110, 113, 115, 119, 131
eosinophilic enteritis 4–5

eosinophilic meningitis 6, 48, 76

Fasciola species 42, 138–40, 142
Fasciolopsis buski 44, 138–40, 144
filarial nematode 29, 59, 63, 72, 130, 136, 141
fish tapeworm 27
flukes
   blood fluke 95
   intestinal fluke 44
   liver fluke 42, 74, 138
   lung fluke 76
fumagillin B 69, 143,

Giardia duodenalis 46, 134, 139–40, 143–5
Gnathostoma spinigerum 7, 48, 133, 139–40, 142–3
granulomatous amoebic encephalitis (GAE) 1
guinea worm 31

haemoflagellate 125
halofantrine 85, 143
Harada culture 51, 105
head louse 78
hookworm 4, 50, 51, 122, 123, 136, 137, 140, 142, 143, 145, 151, 152
hydatid cyst 33–5
Hymenolepis nana 52, 138–40

indirect haemagglutination (IHA) 33–4, 8, 56, 96, 99, 126
iodoquinol 25, 143
Isospora belli 53, 134, 140, 145
itch mite 93
itraconazole 3, 57, 143
ivermectin 5, 60, 64, 73, 94, 105, 131, 141, 143
Ixodes scapularis 13

jigger flea 61
jiggers 61

kala-azar 55
Katayama fever 95, 98–100

ketoconazole 2, 57, 143
Knott concentration 59, 63–4, 131

Leishman-Donovan (LD) bodies 56
Leishmania species 55–8, 134,
   138–40, 142–5
liver fluke *see* flukes
Loa loa 59, 139–40, 142–3
Loeffler's syndrome 11, 104
louse/lice
  body 79
  crab/pubic 81
  head 78

maculae cerulae 81
maggots 61, 62
malarial parasite 83
mango fly 59
Mansonella species 63–5, 139, 140,
   142–3
Mazzoti reaction 72
mebendazole 5, 7, 10, 12, 20, 40, 49,
   51, 65, 119, 121, 123, 141, 143
mefloquine 85, 88, 143
meglumine antimoniate 57–8, 143
metacercariae 42, 44, 74, 76
metronidazole 15, 18, 32, 39, 47,
   120, 141, 143
microfilaria 29, 59, 63–5, 72, 130–2
microsporidia 67, 134, 139, 140,
   142–4
midges 63–5
molluscs 6, 136
myiasis 61, 138–40

Naegleria fowleri 70, 134, 139, 140,
   142–3
Necator americanus see hookworm
nematodes
  filarial nematode 29, 59, 63, 72,
    130, 136–7, 141
  intestinal nematode 11, 19, 40, 50,
    104, 123, 136–7, 141
  tissue nematode 4, 6, 9, 31, 48,
    112, 118, 122, 136–7, 141
neurocysticercosis 110
niclosamide 28, 44, 52, 108, 109, 144

nifurtimox 128, 144
nits 78–81
Norwegian scabies 93–4
Nosema species 67–8

octreotide 22, 68, 144
ocular larva migrans (OLM) 112,
   113
ocular sparganosis 102
Onchocerca volvulus 72, 136, 139,
   140, 143
oocysts 21, 23, 53, 114
Opisthorchis species 74
oriental sore 56
oxamniquin 100

PAIR therapy 34
Paragonimus species 76, 138, 140
paromomycin 2, 22, 25, 38, 47, 144
Pediculus capitis see louse, head
Pediculus humanis (*corporis*) *see* louse,
   body
pentamidine 57, 91, 126, 144
permethrin 78, 81, 94, 141, 144
Phlebotomus species 55
Phthirus pubis see louse, crab
pin worm *see Enterobius vermicularis*
piperazine citrate 12, 144
Plasmodium species 83–9, 134, 139,
   140
  P. falciparum 83
  P. malariae 86
  P. ovale 86
  P. vivax 86
Pleistophora species 67, 68
Pneumocystis carinii 90, 139, 140,
   144, 145
polyhexamethylene biguanide
   (PHMB) 3, 144
polymyxin B 3, 144
pork tapeworm 108
post-kala-azar dermal leishmaniasis
  55
praziquantel 28, 35, 43, 44, 52, 75,
   77, 97–101, 103, 108, 109, 111,
   141, 144
primaquine 87, 91, 144

proglottids 27, 52, 107–9, 138
promastigote 55
propamidine 3, 69, 144
protozoa 1, 13, 15, 17, 21, 23, 25, 37, 46, 53, 55, 67, 70, 83, 90, 114, 120, 125, 133, 134, 141
pyrantel embonate 11, 40, 51, 122, 145
pyrimethamine 116, 145
pyrimethamine-sulfadoxine 85, 145

quinine sulfate 41, 85, 87, 88, 145
quinine dihydrochloride 85, 145

rat lungworm 6
rifampicin 71
river blindness 72
round worm *see Ascaris*

sand-fly 55
Sarcoptes scabei 93, 139, 140, 142–4
scabies 93, 94, 138
Schistosoma 95–101, 138–40, 144
    S. haematobium 95, 138
    S. intercalatum 97, 138
    S. japonicum 98, 138
    S. mansoni 99, 138, 144
    S. mekongi 100–1, 138
Scotch-tape test 40
screw worm fly 61
Septata intestinalis see Encephalitozoon
sheep warble fly 61
Simulium species 63, 72
sleeping sickness 125
slugs 6, 7
snails 6, 44, 76
spargana, sparganosis 102
Spirometra species 102
stibogluconate sodium 57, 145
Strongyloides stercoralis 104, 136, 137, 139, 140, 142, 143, 145
sulfadiazine 2
suramin 126, 145

Taenia species 107–11, 138–40, 144
tapeworm *see Taenia* species

tetracycline 15, 145
thiabendazole 5, 8, 32, 105, 141, 145
thick and thin blood (T+T) smear 13, 59, 63, 64, 84, 86, 87, 126–8, 131
threadworm *see Enterobius vermicularis*
tick 13
tinidazole 39, 47, 120, 145
Toxocara species 112, 136, 139, 140, 142
Toxoplasma gondii 114–17, 134, 139, 140, 142, 145
trematodes 138, 141 *see also* flukes
Trichinella species 118, 136, 139, 140, 142, 143
Trichomonas vaginalis 120, 134, 139, 140, 142–4
Trichostrongylus species 50, 122, 139, 140, 142, 145
Trichuris trichiura 19, 123, 136, 139, 140, 142, 144
triclabendazole 42, 145
trimethoprim 91, 145
trimethoprim-sulfamethoxazole 24, 53, 91, 145
trophozoite 1, 3, 15, 25, 37–8, 46–7, 70, 90, 120
tropical warble fly 61
Trypanosoma species 125–7, 134, 139, 140, 142–5
tumbu fly 61–2
Tunga penetrans see jigger flea

vagabond's disease 79
visceral larva migrans (VLM) 112
visceral Leishmaniasis 55–7

warble fly 61
West African trypanosomiasis 125
whipworm *see Trichuris trichiura*
Wuchereria bancrofti 130–2, 139, 140, 142–3

zoonosis 13, 46, 55, 127